THE CLINIC
TO MANAGED MEN

Norman Winegar

SOME ADVANCE REVIEWS

"This is without a doubt the seminal work on managed care. . . . Winegar's charts and tables make the various models presented realistic. Conceptually, the author addresses the practice implications as well as the critical issues for the future in a thoughtful and searching manner. A truly professional contribution to the development of mental health services, this book is essential in the reading lists of those concerned with delivering and receiving good mental health and substance abuse treatment in the U.S."

Dale Masi, DSW
Professor, University of Maryland

"A survival kit for practitioners in an era when managed care has taken from clinicians the control of their own practices. Those who read and learn from Dr. Winegar's book will survive and prosper. . . . The book provides the practical, basic knowledge required to understand the current revolution in health care and to respond effectively. All this is presented in the clear, concise fashion that is readily understood by the busy, and now somewhat bewildered, clinician."

Nicholas A. Cummings, PhD
Founder and Chair of the Board, American Biodyne, Inc.
San Francisco, California

"Timely and comprehensive. . . . An excellent primer for arming oneself to survive the revolution underway in the mental health and substance abuse care and treatment industry. . . . All stakeholders will find both challenges and guidance in its pages."

Jaclyn Miller, PhD, LCSW
Director of Field Instruction
Virginia Commonwealth University

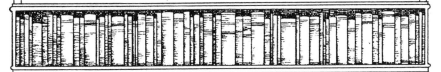

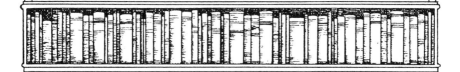

The Clinician's Guide to Managed Mental Health Care

HAWORTH Marketing Resources:
Innovations in Practice & Professional Services
William J. Winston, Senior Editor

New, Recent, and Forthcoming Titles:

Long Term Care Administration: The Management of Institutional and Non-Institutional Components of the Continuum of Care by Ben Abramovice

Cases and Select Readings in Health Care Marketing edited by Robert E. Sweeney, Robert L. Berl, and William J. Winston

Marketing Planning Guide by Robert E. Stevens, David L. Loudon, and William E. Warren

Marketing for Churches and Ministries by Robert E. Stevens and David L. Loudon

The Clinician's Guide to Managed Mental Health Care by Norman Winegar

Framework for Market-Based Hospital Pricing Decisions by Shahram Heshmat

Professional Services Marketing: Strategy and Tactics by F. G. Crane

A Guide to Preparing Cost-Effective Press Releases by Robert H. Loeffler

How to Create Interest-Evoking, Sales-Inducing, Non-Irritating Advertising by Walter Weir

Market-Analysis: Assessing Your Business Opportunities by Robert E. Stevens, Philip K. Sherwood, and J. Paul Dunn

Marketing Mental Health Services in a Managed Care Environment by Norman Winegar and John L. Bistline

The Clinician's Guide to Managed Mental Health Care

Norman Winegar, LCSW, CEAP

The Haworth Press
New York • London • Norwood (Australia)

The Haworth Press, Inc., 10 Alice Street, Binghamton, NY 13904-1580

Library of Congress Cataloging-in-Publication Data

Winegar, Norman.
  The clinician's guide to managed mental health care / Norman Winegar.
    p. cm.
  Includes bibliographical references and index.
  ISBN 1-56024-204-3 (alk. paper) — 1-56024-205-1 (pbk. : alk. paper)
    1. Mental health services — United States. 2. Substance abuse — Treatment — United States. 3. Managed care plans (Medical care) — United States. I. Title.
RA790.6.W55   1992
362.2'0973 — dc20   91-22226
                                                                              CIP

CONTENTS

ABOUT THE AUTHOR

Norman Winegar, LCSW, CEAP is an administrator for MCC Managed Behavioral Care, a CIGNA company. Mr. Winegar has been involved in the managed mental health care field since 1987 and his 14 years of clinical experience have focused on outpatient mental health services, Employee Assistance programming, and substance abuse treatment. He is a frequent presenter at professional conferences and seminars concerning managed mental health care and its implications for practitioners and consumers of mental health services. His forthcoming book from The Haworth Press is entitled *Marketing Mental Health Services in a Managed Care Environment*.

Acknowledgements

This book is aimed at providing counseling professionals and others interested in the delivery of mental health care services to Americans an overview of managed mental health care systems and strategies. It is hoped this book will contribute in some small way to the improvement of services received by American consumers and toward an increased partnership between the payors, providers, and utilizers of valuable mental health care resources.

I would like to thank the following individuals for their contributions and assistance in the preparation of this book: Dr. John Bistline, Dr. Nicholas Cummings, Dr. Ralph Earle, Dr. Larry Hill, Dr. Demetrios Julius, Rick Kinyon, Dr. Dale Masi, Dr. Joseph Steiner, Joseph Strahan, and Susan Feltus who reviewed an early draft of a chapter concerning the legal aspects of utilization management. I am also indebted to the following organizations for their assistance: MCC Managed Behavioral Care, Inc., the National Association of Social Workers, the Employee Assistance Professionals Association, the American Association of Private Psychiatric Hospitals, InterStudy, and Marion Merrell Dow, Inc.

Finally, special thanks to Morelia Ferguson, to Susan Sheridan who helped revise early drafts, and to Eden Alexander who has long supported and encouraged my interest in clinically effective, cost-efficient mental health care.

Introduction

A revolution is underway. It is reorganizing how mental health and substance abuse treatment services are delivered to most Americans. It will have enormous implications for how consumers access and receive these vital services. Moreover, it will affect the practices of all mental health and substance abuse treatment professionals as well as the administrators, managers, purchasers, and sellers of these services. This revolution is Managed Mental Health Care. Though still in its formative stage of development, it has already impacted care across the nation. Its potential to shape the future of the behavioral health care field in the coming years is enormous.

Managed Mental Health Care (MMHC) refers to a variety of systems and strategies aimed at marshalling appropriate clinical and financial resources to ensure needed care for consumers. Its central feature is the heightened activity of employers and insurers in defining what kind and how much care is needed, and therefore, is reimbursable. The revolution promises a practice environment in the 1990s that is radically different from that of only a few years ago. Those professionals who fail to understand these revolutionary changes will see their ability to provide services to their clients and control their professional futures greatly diminished. Those who do understand these changes, and understand that all practitioners in the coming years will be involved in this revolution, will not only exercise more control over their practices and professional lives, but prosper and grow in this era of change. This book hopes to contribute to this understanding.

It is easy to understand the growth of MMHC firms given their demonstrated ability to provide and monitor care while containing costs. Some examples of the dramatic savings these groups achieve for their customers were noted in a recent *AMA News* item (Staver, 1989).

- CIGNA's clients averaged annual mental health cost increases of 6-8% compared with typical 25-30% yearly increases for unmanaged indemnity insurance benefit plans.
- Metropolitan Life reduced its mental health expense by 50% in the first months of its managed care program.
- Aetna reported a savings through MMHC of over $30 million in a recent year.

Not only are insurance companies interested in these systems, but also the large self-insured employers, who have looked to these programs as solutions to escalating mental health benefit costs. In 1990 a bellwether event occurred in the development and acceptance of managed mental health care as a viable employer strategy for containing escalating costs while preserving mental health benefits, when industrial giant IBM introduced MMHC to its vast employee population. It made the move after finding that its costs for mental health and substance abuse care had been climbing at annual rates of 20%, more than double the rate of its health care costs in general. IBM, which already provided Employee Assistance Programs to its workers, contracted with American PsychManagement (APM) of Arlington, Virginia to develop and manage a nationwide network of mental health professionals and facilities. These service providers were prescreened by the MMHC specialty firm. They agreed to offer cost-effective services aimed at the restoration of the employee's normal level of functioning and to participate in APM's utilization management and monitoring program. In turn, IBM's employees and family members were given financial incentives, through their benefit plan's design, to participate in this network of treatment providers.

Other large companies find it equally difficult to manage the costs of mental health and substance abuse treatment services. Like IBM, they too are turning to specialty, managed mental health care firms and processes to contain costs, provide adequate care, and help preserve these important employee benefits. For all of those interested in the delivery of mental health and substance abuse treatment, an understanding of this burgeoning managed care industry is essential. This book will provide the reader with a concise guide to the development, philosophy, and operations of managed mental health care systems. It will inform the reader about trends in this field. It will provide a variety of practical marketing strategies to enable mental health care professionals to take advantage of the many opportunities, while avoiding the pitfalls, presented by this revolution in mental health care delivery in the United States.

Managed mental health care concerns changing long-standing systems and relationships that payors perceive as contributing to the escalating cost of mental health benefits. Traditional health insurance coverage has tended to assure providers and facilities income and revenue through its system of retrospective review of claims, i.e., authorizing payment for services after they have been rendered to the patient and a claim submitted to the insurance carrier. This system provides few incentives for efficiency or cost-effective care: more services provided mean more income for providers and facilities. In this traditional arrangement the patient has maximum choice of provider and facility, while the provider performs the assessment and selects the type, duration, intensity, and setting of treatment. Compensation is based on fee-for-services, with few financial restrictions or barriers to care from the patient's perspective. Largely insulated by the insurance carrier, patients have had little awareness of how this system of indemnity insurance has contributed to escalating health care costs.

Such a system creates anomalies and exceptions to the normal dynamics of a free market economy. For example, as health care costs have risen, the demand for such services has not declined, but, instead, has increased. In turn, the increased costs associated with greater utilization of expensive services have been passed on to employers through higher premiums. (See Table I-1.)

During the 1970s and 1980s, as societal attitudes toward mental illness and addiction changed, insurance coverage expanded to include treatment for emotional and substance abuse disorders. This increased coverage was viewed as increased access to services by the many mental health professionals who had advocated for its adoption. At the same time new provider groups such as psychologists, clinical social workers, professional counselors, marriage and family therapists, and clinical nurse specialists became qualified for insurance reimbursement for their services. These professionals tended to migrate toward the arena of private practice, expanding their practice milieu from the traditional settings of community mental health centers, state hospitals, and nonprofit clinics.

TABLE I-1. Reasons Health Care Does Not Follow the Laws of Supply and Demand

- Consumers don't shop for health care based on price.
- Health care is not advertised by price.
- Health insurance distorts health care prices from the consumer's perspective.
- Lack of universally accepted treatment standards.
- Special nature of patient-provider relationship.
- Consumers lack knowledge about health care services and must trust the provider for treatment recommendations.

Adapted from: William M. Mercer, Inc. (1990). Integrated health plans: Managed care in the 90's. In *Driving down health care costs: Strategies and solutions* (pp. 14-1-14-30). New York: Panel Publishers.

Others shifted practice settings to private, for-profit psychiatric and substance abuse hospitals. These facilities competed for patients with sophisticated marketing techniques and large advertising budgets. They also helped to "increase access" to treatment through the introduction of consumers to their regimen of hospital-based treatment.

Insurers and employers perceived that the same cost escalation dynamic present in health care overall was being replicated in the mental health field. However, mental health care was unique in that it was perceived as a grey area—a field that lacked professional consensus about diagnosis, treatment standards, and expected outcomes, as well as replete with interdisciplinary bickering and friction. Traditional Employee Assistance Programs, early attempts at directing patient care, were viewed as mostly ineffective in addressing spiralling costs in the mental health and substance abuse treatment realm.

The response of these payors for health care services has been to apply the technology of managed care to the field of mental health and substance abuse treatment. The latter part of the 1980s saw the development of this managed mental health care industry, largely servicing Health Maintenance Organizations (HMOs). In the 1990s, MMHC will expand its market to include self-insured employers as well.

MMHC has changed traditional practice in numerous and diverse ways. Most concern increased accountability and structure. Alternative fee and pricing arrangements, the organization provider networks, the hiring of specialized clinicians and clinical managers, the development of practice standards, redesigned employee benefit plans, new models of Employee Assistance Programs, the variety of utilization management technologies and processes, and an emphasis on outpatient solution-focused treatment are only a few of MMHC's change strategies.

As an emerging growth industry, MMHC is frequently a source of confusion and consternation to practitioners, managers, consumers, and purchasers. At its worst, it is perceived as an intrusive, confusing impediment to or interference with clinical practice. At its best, MMHC is a partnership between providers, MMHC firms, and payors in providing quality, cost-effective care to consumers while ensuring that benefits for such services are preserved.

This book will enable the reader to understand the fundamentals of managed mental health care operations, the market for these services, how clinicians and facilities can integrate themselves in the increasingly "managed" practice environment, and MMHC trends in coming years. Appendices provide the reader with useful supplementary information, including an up-to-date listing of the nation's over six hundred HMOs as well as a directory of America's leading MMHC specialty firms.

Throughout this book, the term Managed Mental Health Care, or MMHC, will be used to describe these entities. Alternative, equally appropriate terms such as Managed Behavioral Health Care (MBHC) can be used to describe them or their functions. These firms may provide direct services to clients, provide services indirectly through Provider Networks, or may only manage mental health and substance abuse benefits.

The term "member" is frequently used throughout as the descriptor for the individual consumer of managed care services. "Client" and "patient" are used interchangeably. The term "provider" is a generic one, referencing any practitioner or clinician rendering services.

The book aspires to contribute to the overall understanding of this controversial, growing field by providing information about MMHC systems, their impact on practice in the mental health, substance abuse, and Employee Assistance fields, and how professionals can continue to serve their clients, while prospering professionally in a time of radical change in America's mental health delivery system.

REFERENCES

Mercer, William M., Inc. (1990). Integrated health plans: Managed care in the 90's. In *Driving down health care costs: Strategies and solutions* (pp. 14-1-14-30). New York: Panel Publishers.

Staver, S. (1989, May 26). Employers turning to managed mental health care. *AMA News*, p.1.

Chapter One

What Is "Managed Care"?

Managed care is a term that elicits a variety of reactions from health care professionals. Some practitioners feel anxious, confused, or bewildered as they try to provide traditional care to clients while coping with a maze of acronyms, undecipherable insurance jargon and procedures, and unclear or distasteful "business" concepts that have invaded clinical practice. Others feel resentment or even anger at managed care firms — resentment toward systems that seem to constantly question their clinical judgement and autonomy, and anger toward perceived threats to their professional livelihood. Many clinicians who have fought hard for increased access to counseling and therapy services for consumers are angered by what they see as managed care's roadblocks to individuals and families receiving such care. They point to waiting lists, "gatekeepers" (who may not be clinicians), and excessive paperwork as obstacles to treatment imposed by managed care systems in an effort to restrict or deny services.

Other groups are concerned about managed care as well. Employee assistance professionals, accustomed to directing clients to particular treatment modalities and providers, are now confronted with relinquishing that role to others when managed care systems are involved. Hospital-based treatment staffs face declining admissions, reduced lengths of treatment stays, and radical restructuring of traditional programs due to the influence of managed care. Graduate students in the counseling professions wonder whether or not their education is preparing them for the actual practice environment of the coming decade. Many students and clinicians even question if "private practice" as it has been historically defined will survive in the future. They wonder how and if their "practices" will interface with managed care systems. What new strategies, skills, and innovations will they need to employ to be successful in the era of managed care?

Meanwhile these concerns and questions take place in the larger health care environment in the 1990s — one in which insurance behemoths are purchasing their own specialty managed care/employer services companies; where unions initiate work stoppages over employer benefit issues; where the federal government is experimenting with managed care systems for its CHAMPUS members, while policymakers debate greater federal involvement in controlling health care costs; where consumers are turning to HMOs and other managed health care alternatives as the cost of traditional health insurance products escalate. Rather than wish for a return to simpler times when counseling and treatment services were purchased on a "fee-for-service" basis and client choice reigned supreme, counseling professionals and others are being challenged to learn about managed care systems and how their influence on practice will increase in the years to come. By doing so they will be better prepared to prosper in changing times while fulfilling traditional roles of service delivery and client advocacy.

ESSENTIAL FACTS

Managed care, or, as it applies more specifically to our discussions, managed mental health care, is a term applied to a variety of strategies, systems, and mechanisms that have as their objectives the monitoring and control of the utilization of mental health and substance abuse services while maintaining satisfactory levels of quality of care. MMHC has as its focus the marshalling and coordinating of the appropriate clinical and financial resources necessary for each client's care. Essentially, managed care clients' needs are matched to appropriate treatment resources, and then the delivery and outcome of these resources are monitored. Managed care developed a significant presence in the 1970s and made important impacts in the mental health and substance abuse treatment fields in

FIGURE 1-1. Groups Affected by Rising Treatment Costs

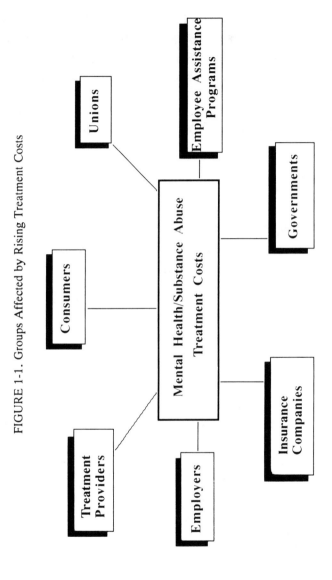

the 1980s. MMHC will revolutionize America's mental health care delivery system during the 1990s.

There are three basic facts about managed care today:

1. *Managed care is here to stay!* It will not go away. Its impact on treatment patterns and reimbursement systems will only increase in years to come. Managed care has already made impressive inroads into the health care market and it continues to grow. According to industry publications, enrollment in America's six hundred-plus HMOs alone grew by 3.9% in 1989, reaching over thirty-five million members by year's end. As the last decade of the century dawned, 14% of all Americans — one in seven — were enrolled in an HMO. HMOs were headquartered in every state but Alaska, Mississippi, West Virginia, and Wyoming. A. Foster Higgins, a well-known employee benefits consulting firm, reported in 1989 that close to two-thirds of employers offered HMOs to their employees. These numbers do not include the millions of consumers who are involved in other types of managed care systems, either through their employers or through insurance carriers.

Some believe that federal legislation may someday do away with managed care through implementation of a national health care system. While the likelihood of enactment of such legislation is questionable due to fiscal concerns, business opposition, and the lack of a national consensus about a "solution" to the health dilemma (including the massive problem of the millions without health insurance who do not qualify for federal and state programs such as Medicaid), such a system would utilize more, not fewer, managed care technologies. By 1990, HMOs already accounted for 25% of the federal employee market, up from 17% in 1987. The reduced costs associated with managed care systems present an appealing option to policymakers strapped with the AIDS dilemma, the costs associated with cocaine and "crack" abuse, and other health-related budgetary problems.

2. *Understanding managed care systems, philosophies, and dynamics is essential for successful clinical practice in the future.* Today more than half of America's physicians conduct at least part

of their practices in association with HMOs. Still others are associated with Preferred Practice Organizations (PPOs). Clearly, managed care systems have exerted tremendous influences on physicians during the last decade, and their influence will extend deeper into the allied health professions in the 1990s. Successful counseling professionals, agencies, and facilities will be those whose practice patterns and programmatic offerings are most attractive to managed care systems.

3. *Managed care is not the problem in health care today.* It is a response to the problem confronting consumers, providers, and purchasers alike: *rising health care costs*, especially that segment of costs associated with the mental health/substance abuse treatment field. To many employers this "grey area" of health care seems particularly in need of "management."

Some estimate that America is presently spending $700 billion per year for health care. Secretary of Health and Human Services Dr. Louis W. Sullivan reported that in 1988 (the last year for which data were available at the time of this writing) the nation spent $539.9 billion on health care, a 17% increase from 1980! Sullivan reported that the nation had resumed its double-digit health care cost growth rate, with an increase of 10.4% over 1987. Previously, the annual growth rate had slowed to single digit increases.

National health care expenditures in 1988 accounted for 11.1% of the GNP, according to the Department of Health and Human Services (HHS). This continues an accelerating trend of skyrocketing costs. (See Table 1-1.) These increases continue to outpace the increase anticipated by the general rate of inflation. In addition to population changes, factors such as utilization of technology, volume and intensity of services utilization, increases in provider charges and spending for hospital services contributed to rising costs, according to Secretary Sullivan.

As Figures 1-2 and 1-3 illustrate, insurance carriers and consumers financed most of the bill for health care in 1988. Hospitals, physicians, and other health care professionals received 80 cents of each health care dollar spent. Tables 1-2, 1-3 and 1-4 illustrate other important aspects of relevant health care cost data.

TABLE 1-1. Percentage of National Wealth (GNP) Spent on Health Care (Reference: *HHS News Release* [1990, May 3]. Department of Health and Human Services)

1960	5.3%
1965	5.9%
1970	7.3%
1975	8.3%
1980	9.1%
1985	10.5%
1986	10.6%
1987	10.8%
1988	11.1%

BACKGROUND: DEVELOPMENTS THAT SET THE STAGE FOR MANAGED MENTAL HEALTH CARE SYSTEMS

Introduction of Prepaid Health Care

Three historical developments helped shape today's application of managed care to the psychiatric and substance abuse treatment fields. First was the gradual development of prepaid health care coverages. The most prominent feature of these systems was that the consumer paid one monthly fee and then received all health care services at little or no cost from selected providers.

Even though the first rudimentary examples of prepaid health care coverage came in the first decade of this century, the major breakthrough for Health Maintenance Organizations (HMOs) occurred in the late 1930s and early 1940s. Industrialist Henry J. Kaiser and physician Sydney Garfield established the first HMOs in

FIGURE 1-2. The Nation's Health Dollar in 1988 (Reference: *HHS News Release* [1990, May 3]. Department of Health and Human Services)

Where it came from....

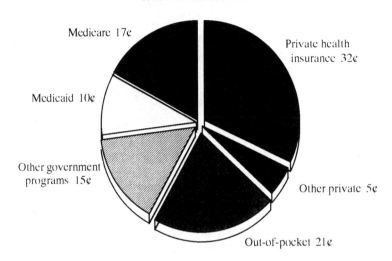

NOTE: "Other private" includes industrial in-plant health services, philanthropy, and privately financed construction.

Oregon and California. They served the health care needs of Kaiser's employees. These organizations were very successful in the cost-conscious World War II era. From these efforts came the Kaiser-Permanente Health Maintenance Organization, the nation's largest group model HMO. (See Chapter Two for discussion of HMOs and HMO models.) Kaiser-Permanente flourished first in Northern and then Southern California. Later HMOs made their appearance in other parts of the country and were particularly successful in the Minneapolis-St. Paul area of Minnesota and in Wisconsin.

Still, by 1970 less than three million Americans in fifteen states belonged to HMOs. The label of "socialized medicine" and the opposition of physician and hospital groups had hampered their growth. It was the Nixon administration who gave impetus to HMO

FIGURE 1-3. The Nation's Health Dollar in 1988 (Reference: *HHS News Release* [1990, May 3]. Department of Health and Human Services)

....where it went

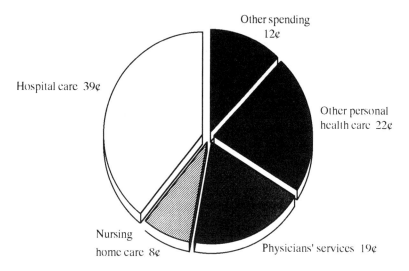

NOTE: "Other personal health care" includes dental, other professional services, home health, drugs, and durable medical equipment. "Other spending" is for program administration and the net cost of private health insurance, government public health, research, and construction.

TABLE 1-2. National Health Care Costs in Relation to GNP and Population (Reference: *HHS News Release* [1990, May 3]. Department of Health and Human Services)

Year	1960	1965	1970	1975	1980	1985	1986	1987	1988
Population (in millions)	190.1	204.0	214.8	224.7	235.2	247.1	249.5	251.8	254.2
GNP (in billions)	$515	$705	$1,015	$1,598	$2,732	$4,015	$4,232	$4,524	$4,881
Expenditures (in billions)	$27.1	$41.6	$74.4	$132.9	$249.1	$420.1	$450.5	$488.8	$539.9
% GNP	5.3%	5.9%	7.3%	8.3%	9.1%	10.5%	10.6%	10.8%	11.1%

TABLE 1-3. Per Capita Health Care Expenditures, 1960-1988 (Reference: *HHS News Release* [1990, May 3]. Department of Health and Human Services)

Year	1960	1965	1970	1975	1980	1985	1986	1987	1988
Dollars	143	204	346	592	1,059	1,700	1,806	1,941	2,124

TABLE 1-4. Average Annual Percent Change in Health Care Costs from Previous Year vs. GNP Percent Change from Previous Year, 1965-1988 (Reference: *HHS News Release* [1990, May 3]. Department of Health and Human Services)

Year	1965	1970	1975	1980	1985	1986	1987	1988
Health Care Cost Increase	8.9	12.3	12.3	13.4	11.0	7.2	8.5	10.4
GNP Increase	6.5	7.6	9.5	11.3	8.0	5.4	6.9	7.9

growth through its support of legislation that "federally qualified" an HMO and mandated its offering to employees in the geographic area it served. Called the HMO Act of 1973, this law required that employers of twenty-five employees or more must offer an HMO option, if an HMO is in operation in their locale, and if requested by the HMO to do so. During the Carter administration, Health Education and Welfare Secretary Joseph Califano simplified the HMO qualifying process and HMOs began to expand. There was a sizable jump in enrollment in the early 1980s and growth continued, though at a slower pace, in the latter part of that decade. The industry as a whole struggled financially during the 1980s as it attempted to control or slow down rising health care costs. Some, mostly smaller, poorly capitalized HMOs failed, while others were purchased or absorbed by larger organizations. By 1990 a financial turnaround had been achieved in the industry. Analysts predict that while the number of HMOs will drop in the 1990s, there will be continued growth in membership overall. Additionally, the success of HMOs spurred the development of other managed care systems such as PPOs which compete for membership (see Chapter Three).

Just as the 1973 HMO Act had far-reaching effects on the development of HMOs, the 1974 Employee Retirement Income Security Act (ERISA) was to facilitate growth of managed care systems as well. Even though this act was primarily aimed at pension equity, ERISA contains a provision allowing self-insured groups to be exempt from most state regulations pertaining to mandated health insurance benefits and mandated provider requirements.

For example, until recently most HMOs charged premiums to employers and employees based on "community ratings," that is, based on the projected cost of services provided to the entire HMO membership, not a single group of employees. Under ERISA, a large employer may choose to fund insurance coverage only for its own employee population. In this way the employer hopes to take advantage of its own efforts to maintain a healthy work force. By not funding and participating in the larger pool of insurance groups, it hopes to achieve cost-savings. Self-insured employers have great flexibility in designing benefits. For self-insured employers, insurance carriers serve only to administer the program. Employers sometimes use Third-Party Administrators (TPAs) for this function, as well. During the 1980s, self-insured employers proliferated. Today, ERISA provisions continue to influence how health benefits are designed and administered (see Chapter Seven for a further discussion of ERISA).

Growth of Private Psychiatric Hospitals

Responding to reimbursement system changes and changes in societal attitudes, the development of private, for-profit, psychiatric and substance abuse hospitals and treatment units was a second factor in the development of managed care systems in the mental health area. These facilities grew rapidly in the late 1970s and throughout the 1980s. The development of the Diagnostic Related Groups (DRGs) as a funding mechanism for Medicare inpatient medical care helped to spur this development indirectly.

In 1975 the DRG system was developed at Yale University and included 467 diagnoses. The federal government began utilizing it for Medicare patients as a cost management tool, a means of sharing financial risk with hospitals. Under a DRG system, a schedule of maximum payments for hospital care is developed for each diagnosis. The hospital is reimbursed for this amount, regardless of the actual length of the admission. For example, if diagnosis "X" is covered for four hospital days, but the patient is well enough to be discharged after three days, the hospital is still reimbursed for four days of care. Likewise, if the patient is so ill that five days of hospital care is required, the hospital will only be reimbursed for four days.

DRGs, a form of managed care, were used for medical/surgical hospital care but were not applied to psychiatric diagnosis, due to the lack of professional consensus about treatment of various disorders. They did impact hospital management by indirectly incenting hospitals to expand into the area of mental health and substance abuse care. These hospitals and specialty units in general hospitals proliferated in the late 1970s and throughout the 1980s.

Another factor that stimulated the growth of inpatient psychiatric facilities were changes in statutes concerning the housing of minors with adults in correctional facilities. As society decided that many troubled teenagers should not be housed in existing correctional facilities, psychiatric hospitalization often became a more attractive and humane alternative (while still fulfilling much of the social control function that was desired by parents and the judicial system). Between 1982 and 1986 the percentage of adolescents as a portion of the population as a whole declined, but the incidence of hospitalization of teenagers went up 350%!

Thus, by the late 1980s, most larger communities had several competing inpatient-based substance abuse or adolescent treatment units providing intensive and very costly care. These hospital-based units became large employers of nonphysician counseling professionals. They marketed toward Employee Assistance Program staff who could direct referrals to them. They also formed lucrative formal or informal arrangements with psychiatrists who were expected to admit their patients to these units for the milieu treatment of the inpatient environment. Often the fees derived from inpatient care became an important income source for psychiatrists, overshadowing their outpatient practices.

Expansion of Counseling Professions

A third development, paralleling the other two, was the proliferation of counseling professions that were licensed by state boards and were reimbursable by insurance carriers. Prior to the 1960s most insurance carriers reimbursed services provided by the nation's relatively small supply of psychiatrists. But during the twenty years between 1960 and 1980, society's attitude toward therapy for emotional and substance abuse problems changed. The number of counseling professions and professionals expanded. Led by the American Psychological Association (APA) and the National Association of Social Workers (NASW), these professions successfully lobbied for legal recognition as providers of treatment services. By 1977 psychology had achieved regulatory status in all fifty states. At this writing, social work is regulated in forty-eight states, while professional counselors have achieved recognition in thirty-three states. Marriage and family therapists and clinical nurse specialists have statutory recognition as mental health providers in fewer numbers of states. Many of these professionals have successfully developed private practices and achieved a broad appeal to consumers. Some promote the "cost-effectiveness" aspect of their respective professions, comparing their charges in a favorable light with those of psychiatrists.

While these professions found popularity among consumers in the 1970s and 1980s, insurance carriers equated the proliferation of providers with increased service utilization and, in turn, increased costs. Insurance carriers passed on these increases, or the risk for them, to the ultimate private purchaser of health care services — employers.

RISK: THE DYNAMIC THAT DRIVES MANAGED CARE

Risk, when used in its simplest connotation, refers to responsibility or liability for payment for services. Before the advent of health care insurance an individual was fully at risk for payment for his or her own health care needs. If the individual had an illness or accident, he or she paid a provider (usually a physician) for the unit or units of treatment received (see Figure 1-4).

With the development of indemnity health insurance and its proliferation during the 1940s and 1950s as an accepted "benefit" of a job, employers took on a large portion of this risk for payment. The employer paid a premium to a health insurance company who then reimbursed a provider (usually a physician or hospital) for care provided to a patient (the employee or family members). This traditional indemnity insurance system maximized consumers' ability to

FIGURE 1-4. The Patient at Risk for Health Care Costs

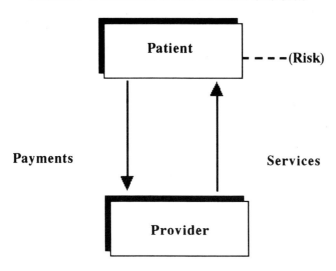

choose the provider or facility from whom they would receive services. It also tended to motivate providers to focus on customer satisfaction while conducting more services, since reimbursement was based on number of services performed. As utilization (number of services performed) grew, insurance companies would periodically reevaluate their costs and charge higher premiums to the employer. As employers purchased policies from insurance companies that included coverage for mental health and substance abuse treatment they took on greater risk for the cost of services delivered by the various counseling professionals and inpatient treatment facilities. In this system, insurance carriers functioned as passive claims payors. Consumers selected the provider while the providers selected and delivered treatment services, which were ultimately funded by the employer through premiums paid to the carrier. Consumers contributed through their payroll deductions and "deductible charges" but employers contributed the majority of the total insurance costs. (See Figure 1-5.)

As health care costs rose in the 1980s, employers increasingly felt themselves in an uncomfortable bind. Faced with a more competitive environment, they struggled for means to contain the escalating impact of health care on their profits, while searching for

FIGURE 1-5. Indemnity Insurance: Employer and Carrier Share Risk

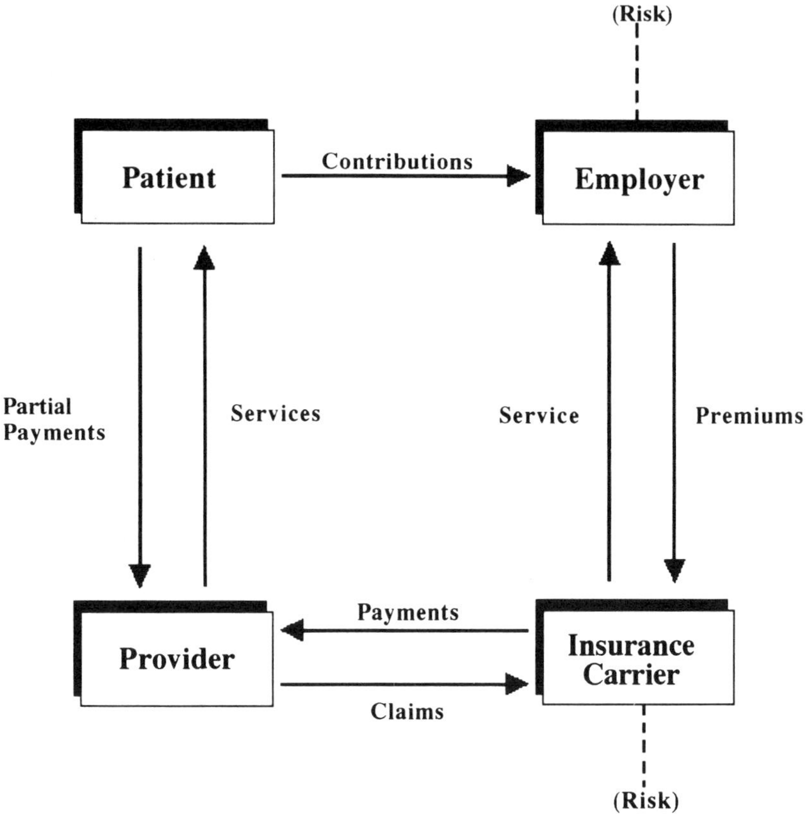

ways to provide adequate care for their employees' mental health and substance abuse treatment needs. Led by IBM in the early 1980s, most of the nation's large employers developed or expanded their Employee Assistance Programs (EAPs). Many, already utilizing managed care in the forms of HMOs and PPOs turned to these organizations as models to address the quandary of how to provide adequate care while containing the escalating mental health and substance abuse care costs. The MMHC specialty firm came into existence to meet this market's needs (Figure 1-6).

FIGURE 1-6. Sharing Risk Through Managed Care

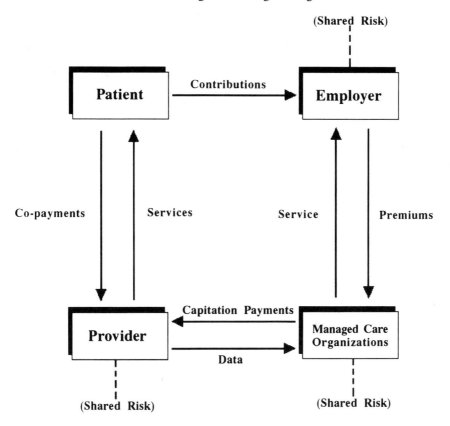

REFERENCES

Bloom, J. (1987). *HMO's: The revolution in health care*. Tucson, AZ: The Body Press-HP Books, Inc.

Califano, J. A., Jr. (1986). *America's health care revolution*. New York: Simon and Schuster, Inc.

Cooper, A. L. (1990). Providers and managed health care. *HMO/PPO Trends*, *3*(1), 5-9.

Cummings, N. A. (1990). The credentialing of professional psychologists and its implication for other mental health disciplines. *Journal of Counseling and Development*, *68*, 485-490.

Garcia, A. (1990). An examination of the social work profession's effort to achieve legal regulation. *Journal of Counseling and Development, 68,* 491-497.

Group Health Association of America. (1990). *1990 national directory of HMO's.* Washington, DC: Author.

Health Insurance Association of America. (1989). *1989 HMO user satisfaction study.* Washington, DC: Author.

Health Market survey. (1990, May 14). Washington, DC: Interpro Publications Inc.

HHS News Release. (1990, May 3). Department of Human Services.

Mahoney, J. (1987, May). EAPs and medical cost containment. *ALMACAN,* pp. 16-20.

Marion Merrell Dow, Inc. (1990). *Marion managed care digest—HMO edition.* Kansas City, MO: Author.

Chapter Two

Managed Care Basics: Health Maintenance Organizations

Managed Mental Health Care systems have been largely derivations of and outgrowths from Health Maintenance Organizations and Preferred Provider Organizations, and MMHC entities utilize many of the technologies, values, and structures inherent in these organizations. Moreover, HMOs represent a major market for MMHC firms, which manage the HMO customer's mental health and substance abuse services. A familiarity with the fundamental operations of HMOs and PPOs provides the background necessary for understanding the developments in managed mental health care.

Health Maintenance Organizations (HMOs) number over six hundred in this country today, and provide health care to thirty-five million Americans. HMOs are large, complex, highly regulated businesses that can operate as for-profit or nonprofit entities. Unlike traditional health insurance carriers, which function largely as claims payors, HMOs both deliver and finance health care. They also differ from traditional carriers in that they provide preventative services and have as part of their focus the "maintenance" of health, not just the treatment of illness. HMO membership grew 10.5% in 1990, a major increase after two years of sluggish growth. Analysts predict HMOs will continue to grow in the 1990s as new products are made available (See Figure 2-1 and Table 2-1.)

The trade association for the HMO industry is the Group Health Association of America (GHAA). It publishes a periodical about the industry called *HMO Magazine*. GHAA's address is listed in the Resource Directory section of this book. GHAA can provide a range of information about its member HMOs and the industry in general.

FIGURE 2-1. HMO Enrollment, 1986-1990 (Source: *Marion Merrell Dow Managed Care Digest*/HMO Edition 1991, p. 7)

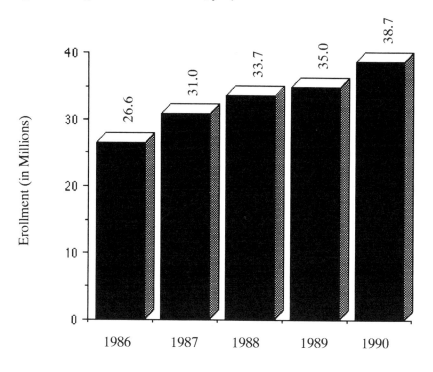

The leading managed health care research and policy analysis institution is the nonprofit InterStudy Center for Managed Care Research (see the Resource Directory for InterStudy's address). InterStudy provides business managers, policy makers, analysts, and clinicians with current data about HMO trends and developments. It publishes *InterStudy Edge*, a widely read quarterly publication.

HMOs provide services (medical, dental, pharmaceutical) to their subscribers, called "members," on a prepaid, fixed fee basis; that is, members pay for services through fixed, monthly premiums. These premiums are usually less than those of traditional indemnity health insurance coverages. (In 1989 average family HMO premiums were $265.50 per month, while individual premiums averaged $99.20 per month.) At the time of service, members may pay an additional charge, a copayment. This copayment is usually

TABLE 2-1. HMO Growth Trends, 1984-1990 (Source: *Marion Merrell Dow Managed Care Digest*/HMO Edition 1991, p. 7.)

YEAR	NUMBER	ENROLLMENT (000)
1984	385	16,784
1985	490	22,660
1986	632	26,559
1987	707	31,024
1988	659	33,715
1989	623	35,031
1990	614	38,707

quite small ($3.00 to $5.00 or so) for basic health care visits or for prescriptions. Copayments to specialists may be substantially higher. Instead of looking to the HMO to reimburse health care expenses that have already occurred, as in the case of indemnity insurance plans, the member looks to the HMO for the actual provision of health care services. Meeting deductibles, filling out and filing claim forms, and waiting for reimbursement checks to come are eliminated. In return for this simplified financial system, members must depend on the HMO to provide adequate access to quality health care services. Figure 2-2 shows how HMOs function, while Table 2-2 contrasts HMO operations with indemnity insurance benefit plans.

THE CENTRAL ROLE
OF THE PRIMARY CARE PHYSICIAN

In medical HMOs the Primary Care Physician (PCP) is the focal point of service delivery. In these organizations, the physician serves as a coordinator (case manager) of health care services, pro-

FIGURE 2-2. How HMOs Function

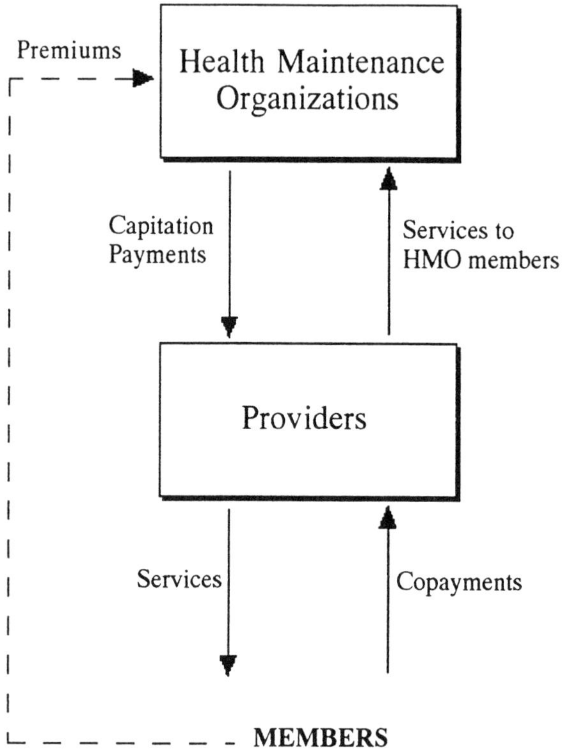

viding care when needed and referring members to others when specialized services are required. His practice serves as the point of interface between the member and all covered health care services. The PCP also functions as a gatekeeper, ensuring that treatment resources are used appropriately. Using his medical judgement and expertise, the PCP determines what type and what level or intensity of care is necessary. (Both these roles, case manager and gate-keeper, are duplicated by specialists in managed mental health care systems as they pertain to mental health and substance abuse ser-vices). In return for the advantages of HMO membership, patients give over to the PCP a degree of choice in health care decisions that is restrained by subscribers to other health benefit plans.

TABLE 2-2. Summary of Managed Health Care Systems

	Traditional Indemnity	Modified Indemnity	PPO	IPA/Network/Group HMOs	Staff HMOs
Provider Panel	Consumer selects any provider	←	Selected providers, with out-of-network choices	Pre-Selected Providers	←
Consumer Choice	Complete freedom of choice	←	Incentivized Choice	No Choice	←
Utilization Review Procedure	None	Precertification of Admissions	MIS Profiling, Concurrent Review		←
Provider Payment	FFS	←	Discounted FFS	Capitation	Salary
Practice Settings	Community-based, independent practice	←	←	Mixed	Clinic Setting
Consumer Payments	Varied deductibles, claims reimbursement	←	Reduced co-payments, claims reimbursement	Co-payments	Co-payments

The way in which physician services are organized defines the HMO model. What follows is a description of how most, though not all, HMOs utilize their physician providers. When a new member joins an HMO, he selects a PCP from the available panel of physicians (usually family practitioners, internists, or pediatricians). Each month thereafter, the selected PCP is paid a fixed, monthly amount for that member and all other HMO members who have selected the physician to be their PCP. The physician then becomes responsible for the provision of all the medical services, preventative and remedial, that were offered to the member by the HMO contract.* Regardless of how much or how little primary care the PCP delivers to the member, he receives the same capitation payment each month.

In addition to the capitation payment, the PCP typically receives an allowance for specialist care, inpatient care, or other referral services. This is called the "referral account." (Mental health and substance abuse care may or may not be included in this account.) The PCP "authorizes" reimbursement for a specialist to provide care, paying for the care through the referral account. That is, the member must first be referred by the PCP before accessing this specialty care. The specialist then submits claims to the HMO, which matches the claim to the PCP's authorization and reimburses the specialist for services rendered to the member. The specialist may also have collected a portion of the charge from the member, i.e., the specialist's copayment. In turn, the HMO credits to the PCP's referral account the amount paid out in claims for specialty care. At the end of the member's contract year, the PCP shares in any surplus or deficit in the referral account. Some HMO systems withhold a portion of the PCP's monthly capitation payments to offset a potential deficit in this account. Also established is an upper limit to the PCP's risk concerning the referral account. The HMO assumes this extraordinary risk which is associated with the unfore-

---

*The HMO's agreement with its providers prohibits billing the member for covered services, affording protection to the member from unnecessary charges. (HMO provider agreements also stipulate an arbitration process for disputed payments. These features are often duplicated in MMHC provider agreements. See the MMHC Sample Provider Agreements found in Appendix A).

seen costs of care for catastrophic illnesses. This risk-sharing system ultimately provides incentive for the PCP to avoid overuse of costly specialty care.*

As an example of how this payment system works, suppose Dr. Smith is paid $10 per member, per month (pm pm). Over the course of one year Smith collects $120 from the HMO for member Jones' primary care. He manages Mr. Jones' and his other patient's care well, so he receives an additional equivalent of $1 pm pm from the surplus of his referral account. His total annual compensation for Mr. Jones' care then is $120 plus $12, or $132. If Mr. Jones visited his PCP three times that year (the average number of physician encounters for HMO enrollees nationally in 1989 was 3.3), Dr. Smith was paid the equivalent of $132 ÷ 3 or $44 per office visit.

As stated earlier, in HMO systems, the PCP is the gatekeeper to health care. He decides when, what kind, and what level of care is needed, as well as its duration. He is the case manager coordinating and monitoring the overall delivery of care. His focus is to keep the member as healthy as possible and to return an ill member to health as quickly as possible. The financial incentives built into the system discourage the overprovision of medical services to the member (in contrast to traditional indemnity insurance, where reimbursement is based on the quantity of services delivered.)

In addition to being care providers, PCPs often involve themselves in various committees within the HMO that help to oversee its clinical standards and operations. Depending on the HMO model, PCPs may see other non-HMO patients as well.

OTHER KEY HMO FUNCTIONS

Aside from reliance on its PCPs for the coordination and management of care, HMOs attempt to contain costs through various alternative payment arrangements with hospital providers. Prominent among these are the use of per diems—a prearranged, negotiated

---

*Aware that patients with prior serious illness may heavily utilize specialist referrals, some PCP's may decline to accept some new patients. This, along with the general unpopularity of specialist refund accounts and withholds among providers, some HMO's are eliminating or modifying such systems.

fee per day of hospital care. By designating a limited number of hospitals as providers, and thus ensuring a volume of referrals for each participating hospital, HMOs are able to receive a per diem rate less than normally charged. Per diems may be negotiated along a schedule, so that if referral volume is lower than expected, the hospital's per diem charge increases.

Another common payment arrangement (mandated in several states) is the use of Diagnostic Related Groups (DRGs). Originally developed in the 1970s for Medicare purposes, this system pays for hospital days based on the respective diagnosis. A patient admitted with diagnosis "X," for example, usually requires five days of hospital care. The hospital is paid for the equivalent of five days of care regardless of the actual length of stay. DRGs represent a form of risk sharing between the HMO and the hospital. HMOs have revised and adapted the original Medicare DRGs for commercial purposes.

Some HMOs pursue discounted fees from hospitals, similar to per diems. Greater volume of patient referrals result in greater discounts from the hospital provider. Another innovative approach is called "bed leasing." An HMO may negotiate an arrangement with a hospital whereby it leases a bed(s). The HMO is assured of access to hospital care in this way, while the hospital is assured of a filled bed(s).

Utilization Management

Another key function of HMOs and other managed care entities is utilization management.* This term describes a variety of techniques and processes that help to ensure the appropriateness, necessity, and quality of care delivered to patients. These processes may be applied before, during, or after care has been delivered. Examples include preadmission certification, case management, concurrent review, peer review, and retrospective chart audits. Utilization management functions are staff intensive and highly specialized.

---

*An in-depth examination of utilization management is found in: *Controlling Cost and Changing Patient Care? The Role of Utilization Management.* Bradford H. Gray and Marilyn J. Field, editors. Institute of Medicine, National Academy Press, Washington, DC, 1989.

(This topic will be more fully addressed in Chapter Six concerning psychiatric and substance abuse utilization management processes.)

Originally associated with Medicare in the 1960s and then with HMOs, these technologies are now widely applied to many indemnity insurance products. This new "Utilization Management" industry, which did not even exist in the early 1980s, has been by and large a spin-off from the HMO field. These firms, the largest of which is Intracorp, a CIGNA company, perform various utilization management functions for the health care plans offered by employers and insurers. Functions include medical/surgical hospital admission precertification and concurrent review. These firms employ nurses and physicians and are typically not at financial risk for services they authorize. Hundreds of these firms operate today.

HMO MODELS

HMOs are usually structured around one of four common models, with some variations. These models are derived from how the HMO structures its panel of PCPs. These descriptions are aimed at giving overviews of how these different HMO models work. (Table 2-3 and Figure 2-3 show the relative enrollments in these HMO models in recent years.)

Independent Practice Association (IPA) Model

IPAs are separate entities from HMOs. Typically they are representative organizations for physicians or other providers who sell their services through the IPA. IPAs may be extensive or very small, encompassing only a few practices. HMOs may choose to contract with several IPAs. Most IPA physicians continue to see non-HMO patients and carry on their own office-based practices.

HMOs pay their IPA physicians on a capitation basis. The IPA is paid a regular fixed amount, usually on a per member, per month (pm pm) basis. In return, the physician who is responsible for the patient's care must provide all necessary and contracted services.

IPAs may form partnerships with more than one HMO, while continuing to provide services to non-HMO patients. Alternatively,

TABLE 2-3. Enrollment in the Four HMO Model Types Nationwide (Source: *Marion Merrell Dow Managed Care Digest*/HMO Edition 1991, p. 5)

	1990		1989		1988	
	Plans	Enrollment (000)	Plans	Enrollment (000)	Plans	Enrollment (000)
Group	77	10,350.0	85	9,844.8	85	8,775.4
IPA	371	16,961.1	386	15,428.0	407	15,138.8
Network	98	7,045.3	86	5,431.5	106	6,163.1
Staff	64	4,350.7	66	4,326.9	61	3,638.3
TOTAL OPERATING	610		623		659	
Developing	4		1		7	
Total U.S.	**614**	**38,707.1**	**624**	**35,031.2**	**666**	**33,715.6**

HMOs sometimes recruit physicians to form an IPA to serve their HMO only, ensuring an exclusive arrangement for that IPA.

IPA models are attractive to HMOs for several reasons. First, they are composed of well-known, community-based providers who usually have existing, successful practices. IPAs tend to be broad-based in terms of service delivery, creating better access for the HMO's members. These factors help in the marketing of the HMO to consumers, an important concern given increased competition. Also IPAs require less capital investment on the part of the HMO than do other models.

However, IPAs do have some drawbacks from the HMO's perspective. The independent nature of the physicians mean their practice patterns are more difficult to influence. Also the IPA represents, in effect, a bargaining unit for physicians—one that can

FIGURE 2-3. IPAs Dominate HMO Industry in Enrollees (Source: *Marion Merrell Dow Managed Care Digest*/HMO Edition 1991, p. 5)

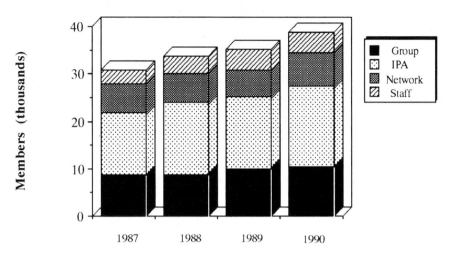

obtain more favorable capitation payments from the HMO as well as other bonuses and inducements.

Staff Models

Staff model HMOs hire physicians as salaried employees. In order to receive covered medical services, members must utilize these physicians as their PCPs. These providers practice in one or more clinic settings. In order to provide the necessary services to its members, staff model HMOs must hire a variety of physicians and specialists. Some contract out specialist and subspecialty services as well as hospital services. Cigna Health Plan in southern California and Group Health Cooperative in Seattle, Washington are examples of large staff model HMOs.

From the patient's perspective, staff model HMOs may seem restrictive. No community-based physicians can be accessed, only the HMO's staff physicians can deliver covered services to members. Some patients object to receiving care in a clinic setting. Such clinics may not be as conveniently located as other physician's offices and there may be more waiting for nonemergency services. Some patients, new to a staff model HMO, may complain at having to form a treatment relationship with a new physician since community practitioners are not involved in this model which is also called a "closed panel."

For the HMO, staff models are easiest to control of all the models with regard to practice patterns and service utilization. This is due in large part to the fact that the physicians are HMO employees and share a practice orientation compatible with the HMO's philosophy. HMO resources normally donated to utilization management may be allocated to other areas or passed along as savings to purchasers. Various economies of scale may also be obtained in such staff clinic settings. On the other hand, the salaries of such large numbers of physicians are a costly expense to HMOs and may negate other savings.

Group Models

Group model HMOs contract with large multispecialty physician groups to provide services to members. These physicians are employees or partners in the group. They share the expenses of their office or clinic operations. They are not employees of the HMO, but rather are compensated through capitation payments. These physicians usually serve non-HMO patients, or may contract with more than one HMO. This is sometimes referred to as an "independent" group model. One of the best known HMOs is the Kaiser Foundation Health Plan which serves over 6.5 million members. It contracts with the Permanente Medical Groups for its physician services. This is said to be a "captive" group, i.e., dealing only with the one HMO's members and resembling a staff model.

Like staff model HMOs, group models give the HMO more control over practice patterns. They also limit members' choices, are "closed panels," and are open to criticisms regarding limited access and "clinic" atmospherics.

Network Models

HMOs sometimes choose to contract with several groups of physicians or independent practitioners to form a broad-based health care network. An HMO may have a panel of numerous family practice physicians, several internal medicine physicians, pediatricians, Ob-Gyns, etc. These systems are called network models. HMOs fund the physicians through capitation payments. The HMO may assist physicians in obtaining discounts from specialists, whom they must reimburse for services the network physician cannot provide. As with other models, if the network physicians provide an excessive number of procedures or make unneeded (and costly) specialist referrals, they will be at a financial loss concerning their HMO patients. Network model HMOs address some of the disadvantages of staff and group models by providing a large number of community-based physicians from which members may select for their primary health care.

INTERNAL ORGANIZATIONAL STRUCTURES

HMOs have boards of directors who have at least nominal responsibility for organizational and fiscal oversight and control. In reality, these boards may exert little influence over day-to-day operations. Boards have differing legal requirements concerning their composition and responsibilities, depending on state regulations.

The executive director or general manager is the key officer in most HMOs. This position provides day-to-day leadership and control over the HMO's operations. This is a CEO type position which supervises the finances, Management Information System, marketing, and other functions. Individuals with educational backgrounds in business, finance, or health care administration are usually employed in these positions.

The other key position in an HMO is the medical director. This officer oversees the various medical management and utilization

FIGURE 2-4. Staff Model

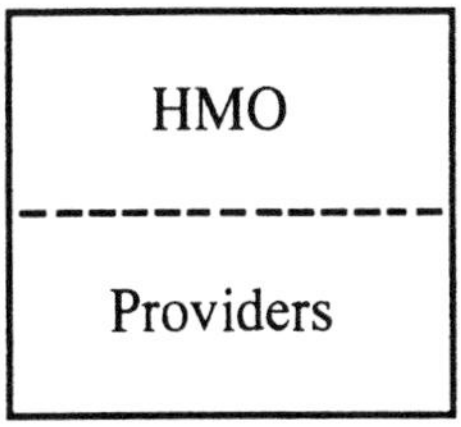

FIGURE 2-5. Group Model

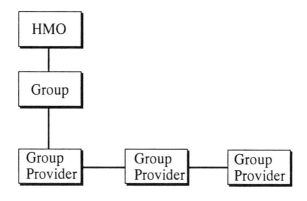

FIGURE 2-6. IPA Model

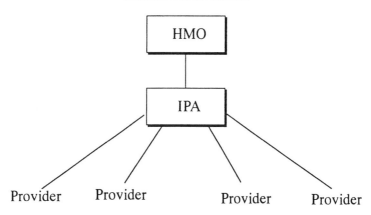

review components of the HMO. This is a complex and diversified position involving expertise in and knowledge of the current state of medical treatment as well as the ability to interact positively with a variety of constituencies. This may be a part-time position in small HMO operations.

Additionally, HMOs frequently have a marketing director, a financial director, and a provider relations director. Staff model HMOs may have a director for mental health/substance abuse services, since this function is provided by the HMO staff.

FIGURE 2-7. Network Model

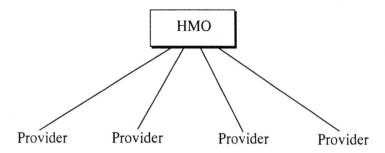

HMOs have departments that process claims, handle member relations, and provide utilization review. Various committees function within HMOs, often chaired by the medical director and frequently involving physicians from the HMO's panel of providers. Examples include a medical advisory committee that reviews which medical procedures should be authorized for coverage; a pharmacy committee that reviews which medications may be included in an approved formulary; a credentialing committee that reviews how new providers are selected; or a quality assurance committee that oversees the HMO's efforts to monitor the quality of care of its members. This last committee may also be the ultimate internal reviewer of member or provider complaints or grievances.

CURRENT TRENDS

HMOs, in sheer numbers, continue to decline, while membership increases. Nationally, HMOs provide health care coverage to 14.8% of the population, according to the *Marion Managed Care Digest – HMO Edition*, 1991.* California ranks first in the nation with over 9.3 million HMO enrollees, or 32.1% of its population. The West Coast states continue to have the highest concentration of

---

*For the recent data concerning HMOs and PPOs contact the *Marion Managed Care Digest* which reports authoritatively about the managed care industry. Write to: Marion Merrell Dow, Inc., Managed Health Care Markets Department, 9300 Ward Parkway, Kansas City, MO, 64114 or call 1-800-3MARION.

membership at 28%. Eleven states — California, Massachusetts, Oregon, Wisconsin, Rhode Island, Hawaii, Minnesota, Arizona, Maryland, Connecticut, and Colorado — have over 20% of their populations enrolled in an HMO. Twenty-four states have at least 10% HMO market penetration. Four states — Mississippi, West Virginia, Alaska, and Wyoming — have no HMOs in operation. HMOs are most successful in the Western region of the United States. (See Table 2-4.)

The HMO market is dominated by its twenty-five largest plans, which together garner over thirteen million (35%) of the thirty-eight million HMO members nationally (1990 figures). Kaiser Foundation Health Plans of Northern and Southern California (the nation's oldest and largest HMOs) continue to exceed two million members each. Other well-known, large HMOs include Harvard Community Health Plan in Boston, Cigna Health Plans (which acquired EQUICOR Health Plans in 1989), and Group Health Cooperative in Seattle.

Table 2-5 and Figure 2-8 describe the market domination by the large HMOs.

Nearly two-thirds of all HMOs were owned by corporations in 1990, a continuation of an upward trend in the 1980s toward corporate control of HMOs. In 1986 only half of all HMOs were controlled by corporations. This trend has far-reaching implications for the industrialization of healthcare.

FUTURE DIRECTIONS
IN MANAGED HEALTH CARE SERVICES

Analysts predict HMO membership, which slowed in the late 1980s, will continue the growth experienced in 1990. The ranks of HMOs will contract in coming years, according to industry watchers, who predict continuing consolidation as underfunded or poorly managed HMOs will not survive. Not even large HMOs seem immune to these financial woes. Maxicare Health Plans, once the nation's largest HMO with 2.6 million enrollees in twenty-three states, recently emerged from Chapter 11 bankruptcy protection. With less than one-tenth its peak membership, Maxicare had entered bankruptcy protection in 1989 with $800 million in liabilities.

Multistate HMO chains, which already dominate the industry,

TABLE 2-4. Summary of HMO Penetration by State (Source: *Marion Merrell Dow Managed Care Digest/HMO* Edition 1991, p. 16, 17)

STATE	1990 Rank	1990 State Population (000)	1990 HMO Market Penetration
California	1	29,063.0	32.1%
Massachusetts	2	5,913.0	28.0%
Minnesota	3	4,353.0	27.7%
Arizona	4	3,556.0	25.1%
Oregon	5	2,820.0	24.7%
Wisconsin	6	4,867.0	21.7%
Colorado	7	3,317.0	21.5%
Hawaii	8	1,112.0	21.2%
Rhode Island	9	998.0	20.8%
Maryland	10	4,694.0	20.2%
Connecticut	11	3,239.0	20.0%
New York	12	17,950.0	18.0%
Michigan	13	9,273.0	18.0%

TABLE 2-4. (continued)

STATE	1990 Rank	1990 State Population (000)	1990 HMO Market Penetration
Delaware	14	673.0	16.9%
Utah	15	1,707.0	16.6%
Washington	16	4,761.0	16.4%
Ohio	17	10,907.0	15.5%
Florida	18	12,671.0	13.2%
New Jersey	19	7,736.0	13.0%
Illinois	20	11,658.0	12.9%
New Mexico	21	1,528.0	12.5%
Pennsylvania	22	12,040.0	11.8%
Missouri	23	5,159.0	11.1%
Iowa	24	2,840.0	10.7%
Nevada	25	1,111.0	9.8%

26	Kansas	2,513.0	9.7%
27	New Hampshire	1,107.0	9.7%
28	Texas	16,991.0	7.7%
29	Vermont	567.0	7.1%
30	Oklahoma	3,224.0	6.9%
31	Indiana	5,593.0	6.4%
32	Virginia	6,098.0	6.3%
33	Louisiana	4,382.0	5.9%
34	Georgia	6,436.0	5.9%
35	Alabama	4,118.0	5.7%
36	Kentucky	3,727.0	5.4%
37	Nebraska	1,611.0	4.7%
38	North Carolina	6,571.0	4.4%
39	Tennessee	4,940.0	3.5%
40	South Dakota	715.0	3.0%

TABLE 2-4. (continued)

STATE	1990 Rank	1990 State Population (000)	1990 HMO Market Penetration
Idaho	41	1,014.0	2.5%
Maine	42	1,222.0	2.4%
Arkansas	43	2,406.0	2.3%
South Carolina	44	3,512.0	2.2%
North Dakota	45	660.0	1.2%
Montana	46	806.0	0.8%
Mississippi	47	2,621.0	0.0%
West Virginia	48	1,857.0	0.0%
Alaska	49	527.0	0.0%
Wyoming	50	475.0	0.0%
TOTAL		247,639	14.8%

Source: Marion Merrell Dow Managed Care Digest/HMO Edition 1991, p. 16 & 17.

TABLE 2-5. The Nation's 25 Largest HMO Plans Ranked by Enrollment (Source: *Marion Merrell Dow Managed Care Digest*/HMO Edition 1991, p. 10)

PLAN	1990 Enrollment
Kaiser Foundation HP/ N. Calif.	2,435,527
Kaiser Foundation HP / S. Calif.	2,277,304
HIP of Greater NY / NYC	905,562
Health Net / Woodland Hills CA	804,561
HMO Pennsylvania/Blue Bell PA	520,050
PacifiCare of Calif. / Cypress CA	485,948
Harvard Comm. HP / Brookline MA	420,767
Health Alliance Plan / Detroit MI	399,960
Group Health Coop./Seattle WA	386,388
PHP of Minnesota/Minneapolis	379,053
U.S. Healthcare / Paramus NJ	376,734
Kaiser Foundation HP/Portland OR	374,451
CIGNA Healthplan/Glendale CA	361,396

TABLE 2-5. (continued)

PLAN	1990 Enrollment
Bay State HC/Cambridge MA	337,341
FHP Intl. / Fountain Valley CA	319,565
California Care/Woodland Hills	312,000
HMO Illinois/Chicago IL	307,236
Group Health / Minneapolis MN	301,360
Blue Choice / Rochester NY	300,993
Foundation HP/Rancho Cordova CA	288,600
Kaiser Foundation HP / Washington DC	279,891
MedCenters HP/Minneapolis MN	261,000
Kaiser Foundation HP/Denver CO	246,706
Takecare Corp. / Concord CA	239,000
Humana Michael Reese HP/Chicago	238,364
TOTAL	**13,561,757**

FIGURE 2-8. Enrollment in Top 25 HMO Plans (Source: *Marion Merrell Dow Managed Care Digest*/HMO Edition 1991, p. 10)

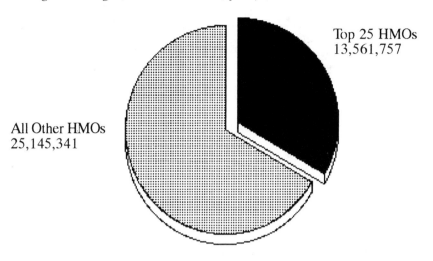

Top 25 HMOs
13,561,757

All Other HMOs
25,145,341

will continue to grow in the 1990s. In 1990 forty-five such companies served over twenty-eight million members, 69% of the total U.S. HMO membership! Table 2-6 describes these chains.

HMOs will increasingly offer new products that afford more choice to members. This strategy, and the products derived from it, will be market-driven as employers in the 1990s will pursue twin goals of cost containment *and* employee service. As the labor pool of capable workers contracts, employers will be increasingly focused on worker satisfaction with benefits programs. In this regard, they will seek increased consumer choice from health care benefit products.

New HMO Products and Services

Open-ended HMO options are increasing in popularity. These plans offer enrollees the choice of using an HMO provider or obtaining care from a non-HMO provider at the point in time that a medical service is needed. These plans are referred to as Point-Of-Service HMOs. A related HMO product features three choices for purchase by consumers: an HMO option, an indemnity insurance option, or a PPO option.

TABLE 2-6. Multistate HMO Companies in 1990 (Source: *Marion Merrell Dow Managed Care Digest*/HMO Edition 1991, p. 8, 9)

COMPANY NAME	# of HMO'S	ENROLLMENT
Aetna Life & Casualty	26	1,290,075
Amer. Health Network	1	20,488
Amer. Healthcare Prov.	2	40,142
Assoc. Group (The)	4	79,400
Blue Cross/Blue Shield	86	4,691,593
Capital Area Comm. HP	6	179,240
CIGNA Healthplan	42	2,228,773
Complete Health Inc.	2	121,900
Coventry Corp.	3	260,392
Exclusive Healthcare Inc.	5	34,023
Family Health Plan	2	121,488
FHP International Corp.	4	559,170
Group Health Coop. (Puget S.)	3	463,016
Health Power	3	27,196
HealthCare Corp. of Am.	3	121,796
Health Svcs. Med. Corp.	2	49,972
Heathsource	4	89,543
Heritage National HP	1	186,858
HIP of Greater NY	4	1,096,948
Humana Health Care	17	981,164
Independent Health	3	252,162
Kaiser Foundation HP	14	6,597,095
Lincoln Natl. Life Ins.	20	473,127
Maxicare HP Inc.	7	284,721
Mercy Alternatives	5	111,696
MetLife Healthcare	26	386,999

COMPANY NAME	# of HMO'S	ENROLLMENT
Mid-Atlantic Health Svcs.	2	257,279
Ochsner Medical Corp.	2	83,420
PacifiCare Health Syst.	5	681,711
Physician Corp. of Amer.	3	109,532
Physicians Health Svc.	2	54,381
Principal Financial Grp.	8	193,317
Prucare (Prudential Ins.)	27	751,863
Qual Med Inc.	10	239,100
Sanus Health Plan	5	626,382
Sentara Health System	2	98,102
Sierra Health Services	1	81,062
Sisters of Providence	3	93,080
The HMO Group	11	1,939,148
The Wellcare Mgmt. Grp.	2	37,217
Travelers Health Netwk.	10	102,984
United American Healthcare Corp.	2	116,283
United HealthCare Corp.	18	1,276,211
U.S. Healthcare Inc.	7	1,092,074
Wausau Insurance	7	71,409
TOTAL U.S.	**424**	**28,653,532**

Another HMO variant, new to the health care scene, is the integrated health plan in which all of a company's employees are enrolled into a single benefits plan. The health care company provides all medical and mental health services to members through its staff or network of providers. Members may be given "opt-out" choices to receive some or all covered services with non-network providers,

HMOs SLOWLY GAIN CREDIBILITY WITH EMPLOYEES, DESPITE LOWER COSTS

Once touted as the solution to rising health care costs, HMOs continue to get mixed reviews from employers. Only 38 percent of a national survey of 1,962 employers conducted in 1990 by the benefits consulting firm, A. Foster Higgins & Co. agreed with the statement, "HMOs are effective in controlling our costs." Twenty-seven percent disagreed; the rest were neutral. Still, this endorsement by America's business leaders was an increase, up from 33 percent who agreed with the statement the prior year.

This less-than-enthusiastic endorsement came despite the fact that HMO coverage cost $2,683 per employee in 1990, 17 percent less than indemnity insurance. Indemnity plans cost $3,214 per employee according to the study. The per-employee HMO cost increase of 15.2 percent in 1990 compared favorably to the increase of 21.6 percent associated with indemnity and PPO plans.

Disenchanted employees will increasingly consider transitioning to point-of-service plans which incorporate the choice dimension of PPOs and the cost containment feature of HMOs, both for medical-surgical and mental health/substance abuse benefits. Such employees will rely upon MMHS firms to develop such services, featuring in-network and out-of-network benefit coverage, for mental health and substance abuse treatment needs. The HMO industry, meanwhile, is rapidly developing new generations of products with these features, many employers offer benefit packages consisting of two options: an HMO choice or a point-of-service, network-based plan. Eliminated will be the traditional, "unmanaged" indemnity insurance plan option.

Point-of-service plans allow covered members to choose, at the "point-of-service," whether to receive care from a network provider (affiliated with a managed care firm) or an unaffiliated provider. Members are incentivized to choose the network provider through increased benefits, reduced out-of-pocket expenses, or the absence of a claims filing procedure. By shifting employee populations into such point-of-service networks, self-insured employers are also able to customize benefit structures, gain a better understanding of their employees' health care utilization patterns, and insure a smaller risk pool, thus taking advantage of employer-sponsored prevention activities such as Wellness Programs and Employee Assistance Programs. Importantly, employers can also ensure that most employees will likely receive the higher quality of care afforded by network-affiliated providers.

A mental health services consumer who selects such a point-of-service plan may access, through a centralized point, via a toll-free 800 telephone number, and request an appointment or referral. The benefit design and cost features encourage the consumer to select a clinician affiliated with the MMHC company.

Alternatively, the consumer may decline the referral, and seek services from a non-affiliated provider, incurring increased out-of-pocket expense or other disincentives, but still receive benefit coverage. Since a network-affiliated provider will likely be selected by most consumers, this development highlights the need for mental health professionals to develop practice patterns compatible with modern reimbursement systems (MMHC companies) and to market services toward them.

Source: Albinus, P. (1991, August 22). Trust: HMOs are gaining it slowly. (*Healthweek*. Vol. 5, No. 16, p. 22.

---

but with increased out-of-pocket expenses and with utilization management provided by the managed care organization.

These health plans can easily be provided by large, national insurance and employee benefit companies to workforces in multiple locations. They can be tailored into various configurations. Since these industry giants can also offer employers other benefit programs such as dental care, vision care, pharmacy networks, workers compensation, claims processing and payment, and Employee Assistance Programs, they are able to truly provide an integrated array of services. These alternatives to traditional benefit programs will seem increasingly attractive to employers interested in cost containment and in simplifying multiple vendor relationships.

SUMMARY

HMOs are complex business structures performing the difficult tasks of both financing and delivering quality health care in a cost-effective way. While several basic systems models exist, no two HMOs are exactly alike.

After rapid growth in the 1970s and 1980s, HMO enrollment has slowed but still continues. During the 1980s, employers and HMOs became increasingly aware that HMOs were not the magic bullet to stop the spiralling costs of health care. Several HMOs have collapsed in recent years with ensuing disruption to members health care and to the affiliated providers and facilities. This contraction of the number of HMOs in operation will continue in the 1990s with enrollment increases, in part due to new HMO products offering more choice to consumers. The field will likely continue to be dominated by a small number of large financial and insurance organizations that have made a commitment to the managed care field and have the resources and management expertise needed for growth and stability.

REFERENCES

Cigna. (1990, June). HMO enrollment at 34.7 million. *Employee Benefits News*, p. 5.

Joint Commission on Accreditation of Healthcare Organizations. (1989). *Managed Care Standards Manual*. Chicago, IL: Author.

Kongstvedt, P. R. (1989). Elements of management control structure. In P. R. Kongstvedt (Ed.), *The managed health care handbook* (pp. 19-23). Rockville, MD: Aspen Publications.

MacLeod, G. K. (1989). An overview of managed medical care. In P. R. Kongstvedt (Ed.), *The managed health care handbook* (pp. 3-10). Rockville, MD: Aspen Publications.

Marion Merrell Dow, Inc. (1991). *Marion managed care digest—HMO edition*. Kansas City, MO: (Company Publication).

Maxicare closes the book on chapter eleven. (1990, December 17). *Health Week*, p. 6.

Mercer, W. M., Inc. (1990). Integrated health plans: Managed care in the 90's. In *Driving down health care costs: Strategies and solutions* (pp. 14.01-14.07). New York: Panel Publishers.

Reynolds, J. D., & Bischoff, R. N. (1991). *Health insurance answer book* (3rd ed.). New York: Panel Publishers.

Wagnor, E. R. (1989). Types of managed care organizations. In P. R. Kongstvedt (Ed.) *The managed health care handbook* (pp. 11-18). Rockville, MD: Aspen Publications.

Chapter Three

Preferred Provider Organizations and Mental Health Provider Networks

Preferred Provider Organizations (PPOs) are entities through which insurance companies or employer groups purchase services for their subscribers or employees. PPOs are organizations, not actual providers. The providers who affiliate with a PPO may be physicians, dentists, hospitals, or nonphysician clinicians. The purchaser, on behalf of its members, negotiates discounted fee arrangements with the PPO in advance of service delivery. In exchange for this discount, employer groups or insurance companies provide incentives for clients to utilize the PPO providers (see Figure 3-1).

HOW PPOs ACHIEVE COST CONTAINMENT

The incentive for members to use PPO providers is achieved through benefit design. For example, the patient who chooses to use a non-PPO affiliated physician or hospital may have benefit coverage for only 70% of the charges versus 90% coverage for the PPO provider. Out-of-pocket costs to the consumer are higher when using these "out-of-network" providers or provider facilities. In this way, all medically necessary services will be covered and the consumer continues to exercise choice over which provider to use. At the same time, benefit design tends to drive service utilization toward the least costly provider (the PPO affiliate), while shifting

FIGURE 3-1. PPO Mechanisms

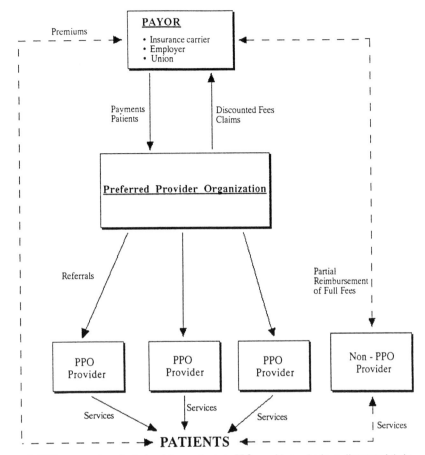

In PPO systems, benefit design drives patients to PPO providers, who have discounted their fees and agreed to utilization management procedures in return for increased patient volume. Patients may still choose non - PPO providers, but the PAYOR will reimburse a smaller share of charges, resulting in more cost-sharing by the patient.

more cost-sharing to the patient who chooses to go outside the PPO network for necessary services.

PPO networks help to achieve further cost containment for the purchaser and consumer. This results from PPO affiliated providers having agreed to cooperate with the payor's utilization management procedures. More about this important feature in the next section of this book.

OTHER FEATURES

A variant of the PPO is the PPA, Preferred Provider Arrangement. This term implies a looser affiliation without an organization. A PPA actually refers only to a discounted fee arrangement between insurance carriers or other groups and a provider or providers. The term "PPO" refers to the organizing entity, but has become more generic over the years.

Another variant of the PPO is the Exclusive Provider Organization (EPO). In these arrangements, services are covered for reimbursement by a payor *only* if services are delivered by a designated provider, group of providers, or a designated facility. There is no coverage for services by out of network providers. Consumer choice in provider selection is severely restricted.

EPOs are utilized by employers or other payors who wish to obtain the greatest cost containment and have the least concern as to the consumer's choice. Due to their exclusive nature, EPOs can discount fees to a larger extent than most PPOs. The increased referral volume offsets the discounted fee structure. Thus EPOs can be lucrative arrangements for cost-effective providers. Like PPOs, Exclusive Provider Organizations participate in or provide other utilization management components. EPOs are more closely scrutinized for quality of service delivery since consumers cannot select an alternative provider if dissatisfied, and still retain needed coverage.

Although both are alternative health care delivery systems, PPOs differ from HMOs in important ways. HMOs take on financial risk for medical services. PPOs assume no risk, as risk remains with the union, employer, or insurance carrier. HMOs are highly regulated through federal and state statues; PPOs largely are not. Finally, HMOs are health care delivery systems. PPOs can be best described as organized brokers of health care services.

PROVIDER SELECTION

PPOs may be general, involving a range of health care providers, or they may be limited to hospitals or specialty areas such as dental, vision, or prescription services. (We will later examine mental health related PPOs or Networks). PPOs can be organized by any of several groups, but focus on the selection of cost-effective treatment providers. Providers that have practice patterns inconsistent with this cost-effectiveness goal are still, at times, solicited for PPO membership. This is done in the hope that the utilization management functions will be able to modify such patterns. Such patterns are more easily discerned today by using Management Information Systems (MIS) to examine a provider's claim submission history.

Providers' documentation of credentials are collected and other administrative data are also maintained by the PPO. Claim submissions are sometimes audited. These steps help to assure quality for consumers and discourage fraudulent practices by providers in the PPO.

DISCUSSION AND TRENDS

PPOs have flourished in recent years as the market pursues the goals of controlling health care costs while providing consumer choice. Industry sources estimate over thirty million American families (seventy million individuals) have access to PPO networks of providers (1989 data). Most become members through their insurance carrier (Johnson, 1990). The financial viability of America's PPOs is difficult to ascertain: Some are subsidized by parent organizations; others operate as loss leaders, in effect; incomplete financial reporting confounds other estimations.

Corporate PPO chains will likely continue to develop in coming years. (Sixty percent of PPO members were covered through the thirty-five largest PPO corporations in 1989, according to the *Marion Managed Care Digest*—see Table 3-1). Another trend is toward the offering of EPO features, especially by PPOs owned by employers and HMOs. PPOs are likely to increase their offering of discounted dental care, chiropractic care, and workers compensation as well as mental health services in the future. PPOs are more likely to focus on the recruitment of cost-effective providers as they

TABLE 3-1. Thirty-Five Largest PPO Chains in 1989 (Source: *Marion Merrell Dow Managed Care Digest*/PPO Edition 1990, p. 8)

CORPORATE NAME/HEADQUARTERS	No. of Plans	Covered Employees
Blue Cross and Blue Shield Assn./Chicago, IL	56	6,736,816
Columbia American Corp./Phoenix, AZ	1	1,449,800
Health Care Compare Corp./Downers Grove,IL	1	900,000
Metropolitan Life Insurance Co./Westport, CT	59	754,959
Occupational-Urgent Care/Sacramento, CA	1	720,000
San Diego Comm. HC Alliance/San Diego, CA	1	625,000
Beech Street PPO/Irvine, CA	1	592,878
Private HealthCare Systems Ltd./Lexington, MA	7	576,000
Prudential Insurance Co./Roseland, NJ	2	535,149
Aetna Life & Casualty Ins. Co./Hartford, CT	4	519,049
Travelers Insurance/Hartford, CT	51	461,235
Amer. General Group Ins. Corp./Dallas, TX	3	389,032
Admar Corp./Orange, CA	7	365,379
Preferred Health Network Inc./Monterey, CA	2	355,496
Transport Life Insurance Co./Fort Worth, TX	1	283,000
August Intl. Corp./Orange, CA	1	260,000
Pacific health Alliance/San Mateo, CA	1	226,118
PPO Alliance/Irvine, CA	1	210,000
Equicor-Equitable HCA Corp./Nashville, TN	28	190,011
Metrocare National Inc./Portland, OR	7	164,995
CIGNA-Connecticut General/Bloomfield, CT	31	163,000
The Hartford/Hartford, CT	3	156,286
Capp Care Inc./Fountain Valley, CA	90	150,000
Health Risk Management/Minneapolis, MN	1	143,500
Mass. Mutual Life Ins. Co./Springfield, MA	27	141,629
Intergroup Services Corp./Radnor, PA	1	130,000
Interplan Corp./Stockton, CA	1	120,000
Sisters of Providence/Seattle, WA	2	116,955
General American Life Ins. Co./St. Louis, MO	1	108,082
Medical Control Acquisition Corp./Dallas, TX	1	103,000
Self-Labor Trust Fund/Newark, NJ	1	100,000
Humana Health Care Plans/Louisville, KY	20	97,005
New York Life Insurance Co./New York, NY	1	80,000
United Northwest Services/Spokane, WA	1	75,000
John Hancock/Boston, MA	5	71,362
TOTAL	421	18,070,736

become increasingly aware of practice patterns through better management information systems and technologies. Owners of PPOs will likely confront practitioner opposition to exclusion from networks and will also continue to oppose increased regulation of the industry.

POINT-OF-SERVICE NETWORKS

An emerging trend in employer-sponsored health care benefits is a variant of the PPO, the Point-of-Service (POS) network. According to some, POS networks unite the best features of traditional indemnity insurance with the HMO philosophy. POS networks offer a choice to their members who may, *at the point of service*, choose to utilize a network provider or a non-network provider. By choosing the network provider the consumer enjoys richer benefits, lower out-of-pocket expenses, and reduced paperwork such as completing claim forms. The health care plan still provides coverage for non-network services, but with increased cost-sharing, reduced benefits, etc. Many large employers have come to view these POS network plans as a palatable first step into the managed care realm—one that preserves choice and yet through cost-sharing helps employees become more aware of the actual cost of health care. Table 3-2 illustrates a sample benefit summary associated with a POS network.

Though not affording absolute reductions in health care costs to employers, POS networks are often able to slow rising costs and help employers better predict costs. This due to the inherent qualities of a coordinated network of providers working together to manage patient care. Case management helps to reduce the duplication of services and discounted fee arrangements negotiated by the POS managers with network providers also helping to reduce cost increases to purchasers. Quality management programs are used to evaluate outcomes and monitor the care delivered.

TABLE 3-2. Sample POS Network Benefits: Medical/Surgical

In-Network Benefits	Out-of-Network Benefits
• Most services covered 100% after small co-payment	• Most services covered at 80% level
• No deductible	• Deductible = $300 for an individual, $600 for a family per year
• Out of pocket maximums $500/$1,000	• Out of pocket maximums $3,000/$6,000

- Preventative services
  available

- No claims forms
  to file

- Pre-certification is
  automatic, i.e. provided
  by the network and is
  transparent to the participant

- No preventative service
  available

- Participant must file
  claims forms

- Participant is responsible
  for contacting
  pre-certification entity

MENTAL HEALTH PROVIDER NETWORKS

Employers increasingly view the delivery of quality mental health services to their workforces as an important, but costly endeavor. Noting that as few as five percent of their employees' claims (those with mental health or substance abuse diagnoses) often account for as much as 25 percent of the company's health care expenditures, large self-insured employers are turning to this variant of the POS network as a means of delivering mental health services to their workforces. Managed mental health care firms, eager to expand their market beyond HMOs, have quickly responded by organizing and managing networks of mental health and substance abuse providers and facilities to serve the "employer market."

MMHC network managers provide case management, utilization reviews, and other services discussed elsewhere in this book, that help to control costs and ensure quality care. These networks may be offered in conjunction with employer-sponsored Employee Assistance Programs, which are sometimes also delivered by the MMHC firm. Some employers design such services to function as the assessment entity while the network of mental health providers offer treatment services. Network managers screen, accredit, train, and monitor the performance of network-affiliated providers.

For consumers, incentives are structured into these benefit designs that motivate them to utilize network providers. As with POS networks, features such as enriched benefits, reduced out-of-pocket expenses, and little or no paperwork achieve this end. Many mental health provider network benefit plans provide for coverage even if the employee chooses to select a non-network provider for care (see Table 3-3).

TABLE 3-3. Sample POS Network Benefits: Mental/Substance Abuse

	In-Network	Out-of-Network
Deductible	$0	$300/600
Out-of-Pocket Maximums	$500/1,000	$3,000/6,000
Lifetime Maximums	$500,000	$50,000
Hospital Confinement Limits	None (Length of care is based on medical necessity)	30 day/year 2 substance abuse confinements per lifetime
Inpatient Coverage per Admission	100% after $100	80% after the deductible
Outpatient Coverage per Office Visit	100% after $10 100% after $5 (group therapy)	50% after the deductible

These systems also offer convenience, since the employee need only dial a toll-free telephone number to access either emergency or routine care through the network. Eligibility for coverage of needed mental health services may be accomplished quickly at this juncture. The MMHC staff then monitor and manage both the financial (i.e., paying the provider's claims or bills) and clinical resources needed to address the patient's needs. In mature, smoothly functioning networks activities such as concurrent reviews are conducted on a collegial basis between clinicians who manage the network and the clinicians who provide the care. In new or overly inclusive networks, this may not be the case however. In these scenarios providers, seeking referrals, may join a network only to find that they do not have the skills, clinical orientation, or efficiency in practice to be a successful network provider in a MMHC system. This may lead to disagreements and complaints and even the involvement of the patient in the dispute. (Refer to Chapter Five for a full discussion of MMHC core functions.)

These mental health provider networks developed to serve widespread employee populations along with managed care systems serving growing HMO populations represent the evolving trend in the mental health care delivery system in the 1990s. As their prevalence increases the implications for mental health clinicians and facilities are enlarged. A thorough understanding of the clinical and administrative dynamics and processes of these MMHC systems is essential for professionals serving America's mental health needs.

REFERENCES

Cigna. (1990, November). Preserving products attractive to customers. *Managing Integration*, pp. 1-3.

Marion Merrell Dow, Inc. (1990). *Marion managed care digest—HMO edition*. Kansas City, MO: Author.

Reynolds, J. D., & Bischoff, R. N. (1991). *Health insurance answer book* (3rd ed.). New York: Panel Publishers.

Wagnor, E. R. (1989). Types of managed health care organizations. In P. R. Kongstvedt (Ed.), *The managed health care handbook*, (pp. 11-18). Rockville, MD: Aspen Publishers.

Chapter Four

Employee Assistance Programs: Integrating Managed Care Functions

Employee Assistance Program (EAP) refers to employer-sponsored counseling and intervention services aimed at assisting employees with substance abuse, mental health, legal, financial, family, or other problems that impact worker productivity or safety. Estimates are twenty thousand EAPs exist today, employing thousands of counseling professionals. Leading national providers of EAPs include Personnel Performance Consultants (PPC), Human Affairs International (HAI) (a recently acquired division of Aetna, the insurance and financial services company), and MCC Managed Behavioral Care, (a CIGNA company).

Historically, EAPs have had dual purposes: aiding the individual to overcome personal problems that affect workplace performance and assisting the employer to have a healthier, more productive labor force. Many employers are adding another dimension to their EAPs' tasks, that of helping to manage mental health care benefits. This challenge offers EAPs new opportunities as well as threats. It promises to transform traditional EAPs.

"This is a crucial time for the EAP field," says Dr. Dale Masi, president of Masi Research Consultants in Washington, DC and a professor of social work at the University of Maryland (Personal communication, 1990). Masi, one of the pioneers in the EAP work field, believes these programs are in danger of being swept away as MMHC systems take over many functions once associated with EAPs. "It's up to EAPs themselves to respond to this challenge and find their future identity," Masi says. She believes this will involve EAP professionals in more managed care functions.

EAPs have always had as part of their function the assessment (role induction and diagnosis) of MH/SA problems and referral (determination of the most appropriate treatment resource). EAPs have also provided monitoring and follow-up (case management) for their clients' progress. These are key managed care tasks as well, although many in the EAP field have been slow to recognize the similarity to MMHC systems. Many EAP professionals have been averse to wearing any sort of managed care label, and instead have opposed and resisted managed care technology, viewing managed care as an intrusion and an impediment.

Understanding the ways that these tasks, which are only a small part of overall EAP services, are managed care functions is important. A core philosophy in the managed care arena is that an accurate diagnosis leads to proper treatment. An independent EAP (or Managed Care) assessor who is not affiliated with any treatment facility or group may eliminate any economic incentive to refer to a particular provider or institution. Referral to an appropriate level of care may be based solely on clinical presentation. Contrast this with some facilities which, for example, provide "free assessments" but who usually refer assessed patients to their own services. These assessments then become a community relations vehicle and a means of role induction for the prospective patient.

Another example of economic incentives biasing accurate assessment of patient needs is the EAP marketed by some hospitals. While offered at a substantial discount, many employers have found they are not such a bargain after all, since these EAP counselors may inappropriately refer employees to their hospital's inpatient setting when the patient could have been equally well served on an outpatient basis. Thus an accurate diagnosis established by EAP professionals, as within managed care systems, can lead to patient referral to an appropriate level of care and treatment setting, while avoiding referrals based on economic incentives.

Finally, properly qualified EAP staff may provide the case management services offered by MMHC specialty programs. These case managers both monitor the clinical services provided and authorize benefits to pay for the cost of services.

The evolution of MMHC systems has witnessed many of these EAP related functions, as well as others assumed by the staff of the MMHC organization or by other providers. Employers are reexamining what their EAPs are achieving, at what cost, and how they can be integrated with MMHC functions or organizations. Some think that EAP programs and staff will fail to respond to MMHC and will largely disappear as a separate entity in the coming years, unless they integrate managed care philosophies and functions. How they can achieve this while retaining their valuable qualities of service and advocacy in the business environment of the 1990s represents EAP's greatest challenge.

BACKGROUND AND DEVELOPMENT

EAPs have their origin in early twentieth century employer-sponsored counseling services. Staffed with nonprofessionals, these early efforts were inspired by the Temperance movement. They aimed at helping employees with alcohol abuse and its resulting family problems. The first such program was established in 1917 by Macy's Department Store in New York City. The field of occupational social work traces its origin to these early efforts by employers to intervene with troubled workers. Such programs were boosted by the Alcoholics Anonymous movement in the 1930s and particularly by World War II. During the War, worker productivity and safety was important to national security and more employers instituted these programs. They were then called Occupational Alcoholism Programs (OAPs), a term that persisted into the 1970s. One of the most prominent was that of Kaiser Shipbuilding, one of the companies owned by industrialist Henry Kaiser, the pioneer of Health Maintenance Organizations. Allis-Chalmers, Consolidated Edison, Illinois Bell, and Kodak also established these programs. Union involvement in EAPs dates to this era. After the War, interest declined and during the prosperous 1950s fewer than fifty programs functioned nationwide.

The EAP movement became reenergized in the late 1970s with America's new recognition that substance abuse and psychiatric problems were widespread and were creating much human suffering as well as affecting our productivity and national competitiveness. OAPs changed into EAPs, the name change reflecting the new "broad brush" approach. Their focus expanded to include identifying and assisting workers with problems other than alcohol abuse.

The military recognized the need for such services in the 1970s as well, and the U.S. Navy's EAP became a prototype. America's heightened consciousness of substance abuse problems and the enactment of the Drug Free Workplace Act in the late 1980s added further momentum to EAP development.

Ironically EAPs did not take advantage of an opportunity in the 1980s to supplant the managed care industry. Had the EAP field better focused its energy and resources on the management of both the clinical and financial resources needed for the care of employees, the managed care industry may not have mushroomed in the late 1980s. Inflexible views about the role of the EAP, lack of identity as a profession, inadequate training, and other issues prevented the EAP community from assuming the role played by managed care systems. In fact, some employers came to question whether or not their EAPs' referral patterns were actually escalating health care costs needlessly.

Today there are well over twenty thousand EAPs, large and small, most of which have been implemented in the last ten years. Most all the Fortune 500 companies have such programs, as do many governmental bodies, some unions, and large numbers of small to medium-sized employers.

HOW EAPs WORK

The central task of an EAP is the early detection, assessment, and amelioration of worker problems that affect productivity. Toward this goal, EAPs have traditionally had the following basic components, which are also described in Figure 4-1.

- *Consultation/Policy Development.* EAP staff are technical support to human relations and other managers in developing policies concerning substance use/abuse, as well as other worker behavioral problems and issues.
- *Training.* EAPs provide information to front line supervisors, managers, and union personnel about how to identify, document, and refer troubled workers to the EAP.
- *Prevention and Awareness Activities.* EAPs aim to publicize

their services to employees, thereby attracting voluntary referrals, or in helping employees prevent problems.
- *Assessment and Referral.* EAP staff interview troubled employees and refer them to treatment or other resources. They
provide follow-up monitoring of the case until the problem is
resolved. This may be coordinated with the company's supervisors or managers.
- *Statistical Reporting.* EAPs collect and report various aggregate data to the employer about the utilization of services.

Referrals to EAP counselors may be voluntary, that is, initiated
by the worker or dependent without any coercion from the company. Alternatively, a supervisor may identify a deficit in work
performance and suggest or mandate EAP use as a means of addressing the job performance difficulty. Positive results from drug
screens may also result in mandatory EAP referrals. These cases,
called supervisory or mandatory referrals, involve job jeopardy and
its obvious legal ramifications. They require close coordination between EAP staff, the employer, and treatment resources. Confidentiality is stressed in either case, and information reported to supervisors is limited to essentials and provided within the normal bounds
of disclosure processes. Figures 4-2 and 4-3 show the client flow in
EAPs.

For our discussion, the key aspect of traditional EAP services is
that EAP staff assess when and what type of treatment service is
needed and select an appropriate treatment resource or provider.

BASIC DELIVERY SYSTEMS

The above EAP functions can be carried out in one of several
delivery systems. Here are some of the most common ones.

Consortium. Several employers join together to develop a common EAP entity for their respective employees. Costs are shared.
This arrangement often makes EAP services available to small employee groups that otherwise would not have such a program. Industrial or office parks are typical settings for consortiums. EAP
staff are directly or indirectly employees of the consortium.

Network. Employers utilize a centralized EAP staff, which ar-

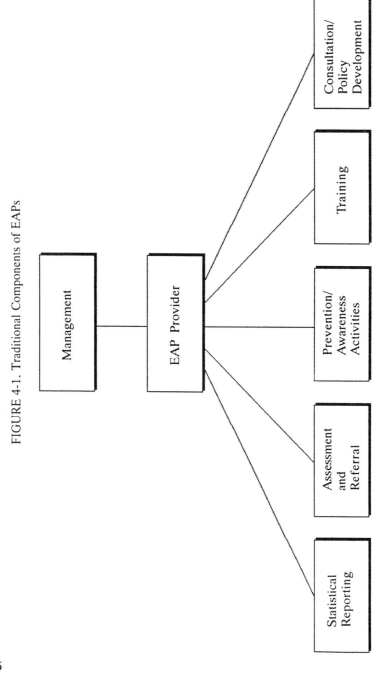

FIGURE 4-1. Traditional Components of EAPs

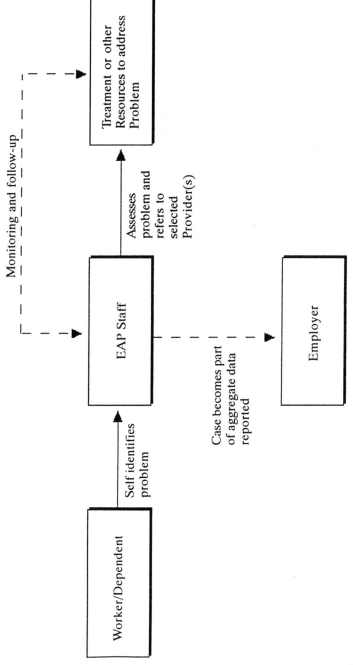

FIGURE 4-2. Voluntary Referral Flow Chart

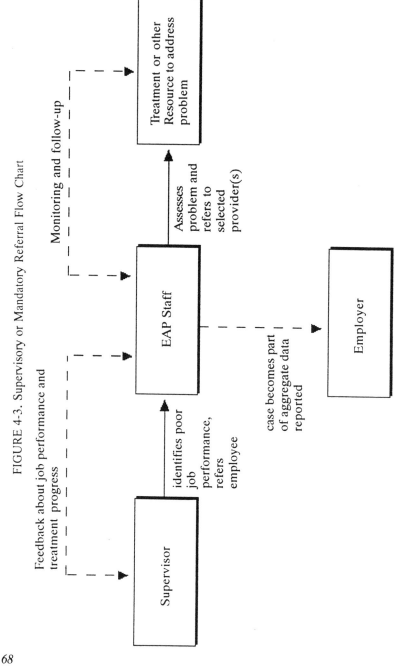

FIGURE 4-3. Supervisory or Mandatory Referral Flow Chart

Feedback about job performance and treatment progress

Monitoring and follow-up

Treatment or other Resource to address problem

Assesses problem and refers to selected provider(s)

EAP Staff

case becomes part of aggregate data reported

Employer

identifies poor job performance, refers employee

Supervisor

ranges training, consultation, and local assessment and referral services through a network of contractors or "affiliates." Access to initial telephonic screening is provided by 800 numbers prior to referral for further assessment. This is a type of external program. Employers with widely dispersed employee populations often utilize such models. These programs are sometimes criticized as impersonal or detached due to a perception of overreliance on telephonic screening and intake services.

In-House or Internal Programs. Employers hire EAP staff that usually function out of the company's medical department. In essence, the company "builds" its own program, usually providing assessment and referral services on site. Staff are extremely familiar with the company and its workforce. These programs must work to overcome the negative impact on utilization frequently brought about by worker distrust based on perceptions that the staff are too closely associated with company management. (Unions may "build" similar programs for their members in one or more workplaces and face analogous distrust by management.)

External Programs. A generic term referring to various programs developed by EAP firms and sold to companies or other employers. Services may be provided on or off the work site. Most programs today are of this type.

EAP STAFFING

A general trend in the field has been one of increasing professionalization. With its alcoholism-specific focus, the early OAPs and EAPs often utilized recovering employees, transferred from their original positions to work in or help develop the service. These individuals, trained in counseling essentials, were basically peer counselors — employees who had achieved sobriety, were involved in the self-help community, and could easily relate to those likely to use the EAP.

With the advent of broad-brush EAPs in the 1970s and 1980s, staffing needs shifted. Individuals with broader counseling and assessment skills were required. Clinical social work, with its history of interest in services delivered occupational settings, has been heavily drawn upon for EAP staffing needs. Psychologists, substance abuse counselors, and psychiatric nurses are also well-represented in EAP positions. Superior salaries and good working conditions have made EAP staff positions attractive to many (Bennet et al., 1989). The number of professionals employed directly or indirectly in the field is not known, but may range into the tens of thousands.

In the late 1980s, the Employee Assistance Professionals Association (formerly ALMACA), which represents some six thousand members, initiated the Certified Employee Assistance Professional (CEAP) credential. This credential does not have an educational standard, but instead it is awarded to individuals with EAP work experience who pass a competency-based test. Presently there are over twenty-five hundred holders of the CEAP credential.

There are no professional degree programs in "EAP." Numerous workshops and seminars offer EAP training and CEU credits. The School of Social Work at the University of Maryland offers a specialization EAP work for its MSW students. But it is unlikely that academia will soon start formal degree programs in this field. According to Dale Masi, a social worker who founded the University of Maryland's EAP specialization tract, many schools are waiting to see what the future holds for EAP, particularly whether or not its functions will be integrated into managed care systems and EAP lost as a potential field of study in and of itself.

DO EAPs CREATE A RETURN ON INVESTMENT?

There has always been discussion about the extent of savings to employers achieved through their EAPs. Cost savings can be measured by evaluating data from several areas. Some areas lend themselves to quantification much more easily than others, while changes in some categories of data cannot be easily attributed to effective EAPs.

Data pertaining to medical claims costs (employee/family) and turnover rate due to MH/SA problems are easy to quantify and relate to EAP effectiveness. This is not the case, however, for data pertaining to overall workforce turnover, absenteeism, sick days, workforce morale, grievances, and on-the-job-accidents.

Some internal EAPs have produced excellent studies of their cost savings to employers. McDonnell Douglas Corporation, disappointed with its EAP's performance, restructured the program in 1985. It asked its consulting firm, Alexander and Alexander, to evaluate the financial offset of the revitalized program. Over a four year study period, Alexander and Alexander reported substantial savings through the EAP, as much as a 35% reduction in medical claims costs (McDonnell Douglas Corporation Employee Assistance Program Financial Offset Study 1985-1988. D. C. Smith, Director, EAP, McDonnell Douglas Corporation, Personal Communication, Sept. 1990.)

Most employers and EAP providers have not produced studies such as this. However there is general agreement among employers that EAPs are valuable tools that serve many purposes. Many employers feel EAPs help avoid the unnecessary litigation of unlawful discharge suits brought about by dissatisfied former employees, terminated for job difficulties related to personal problems. Also EAPs are increasingly perceived as yet another important mechanism available to management to develop and maintain a healthy workforce. They are also viewed as a key employee benefit.

FUTURE TRENDS

Like all other aspects of clinical practice, the development of managed care organizations presents both challenges and opportunities to EAPs. It is likely that EAPs will continue their evolutionary course, incorporating new and expanding upon existing managed care functions. An alternative scenario is that MMHC will incorporate EAP functions into existing managed care technologies and systems effectively eliminating the EAP field as an independent and separate entity.

How have professionals within the EAP field responded to MMHC? Most have hardly welcomed it. Many EAP professionals, long accustomed to making decisions about which treatment resources to utilize, find this role negated or preempted by MMHC and have reacted angrily against managed care systems, often under the rubric of client advocacy. Many have expressed valid concerns about the operations and philosophy of some MMHC systems. Others have encouraged colleagues to take up the mantle of managed care and extend their scope of practice into this new practice area.

For example, Lee Wenzel, a consultant for Managed Care Systems in Eden Prarie, Minnesota encourages EAP professionals to take an aggressive course in building on their case management expertise and expanding the role into both clinical and financial management of services. Wenzel also believes EAPs can take over administrative duties provided by MMHC or Third Party Payors (TPAs). These tasks include eligibility (for benefits) determination, verification of diagnosis, and even claims adjudication and payment. Wenzel states that "EAPs are still one of the best examples of managed care, if only we knew it and believed it. . . . We need to cherish our heritage and grow from it" (Wenzel, 1990).

These views have been recently echoed by the field's professional organization, EAPA (see Dolan, "Development of MMHC Services is an EAP's Best Bet for Longevity," July, 1990 EAPA Exchange). While a major focus of this organization in the last decade has been the ongoing task of legitimization and professionalization of the field, it has addressed the MMHC issue in ways similar to other professional associations. Task forces have been formed to study the matter. Continuing education activities have been offered on the topic. Some groups have even made efforts at developing treatment standards that would guide referral and level of care decisions. Undoubtedly MMHC will continue to be an issue vital to EAPA.

Meanwhile, how are employers reassessing their EAPs and the need for them? Table 4-1 is a list of questions that benefit managers, human resource staff, benefit consultants, and others may find useful concerning how to evaluate the capacity of EAPs to integrate MMHC functions.

TABLE 4-1. Questions for Benefit Managers, Benefit Consultants and EAP Administrators to Consider Concerning Adding MMHC Components to EAPs

Concerning Clinical Service Delivery
- What clinical services are presently being delivered through the EAP?
- How does the organization wish to expand clinical services?
- What are the costs associated with expanded services, i.e., staffing, offices, etc?
- Which services should be added? Extended Treatment Component, Concurrent Review? Precertification? A Provider Network? After Hours Crisis Intervention?

Concerning Staff and Program
- What are the staff's credentials and training?
- Can existing staff perform increased clinical services?
- Is more training needed for EAP staff? At what cost?
- Will EAP staff need more clinical supervision with additional clinical duties? At what cost?
- Does the program provide 24-hour access?
- How can its information system accommodate added functions?
- Can the program function as a TPA?
- What is the EAP staff's level of sophistication concerning managed care technology?
- Can the staff provide meaningful consultation to the organization about MMHC technology and implementation?

Concerning the Referral Network
- How formalized is the EAP's referral network?
- Are discounted fee arrangements involved?
- Is the existing network cooperative with utilization management procedures?

Regarding Referral Patterns
- What is the referral pattern of the EAP?
- — use of outpatient resources?
- — use of inpatient resources?
- is inpatient care being overutilized by the EAP? If so, why?
- Does the staff seem to overutilize one particular provider or institution? Why?
- Does the EAP staff accept renumeration from referral resources or individuals?

Regarding Staff
- What is the level of training of existing staff?
- Are existing staff qualified and credentialed to treatment services?
- Would additional professional supervision be required if staff perform treatment services?

General
- Has the EAP been evaluated by an independent third party with appropriate resources and sophistication concerning both EAP and MMHC systems?
- Does the organization presently understand the MH/SA benefit utilization and claims costs?
- Can benefits be redesigned to support an EAP with managed care aspects?
- There is general agreement that EAPs are important components of the overall benefit/human resource mix and that they save money. Can the existing EAP be retooled and redesigned to include MMHC functions, thus increasing savings, eliminating duplications, and improving client service?

EAP RETOOLING

With the dwindling skilled workforce in the 1990s, employers will increasingly turn to Employee Assistance Professionals for input about and management of various employer-sponsored services aimed at promoting and maintaining a healthy, stable workforce. EAP staff will find themselves involved in developing or consulting about the development of child care, elder care, health promotion, and worker education and training services. These programs and functions may become customary components of future EAP models of service delivery. But employers will also look to EAPs for help in meeting the twin goals of providing for their employees' mental and emotional health needs while containing or restraining the rising cost associated with providing these treatment services.

Employee Assistance Professionals may respond to this portion of their challenge in the 1990s by developing an EAP with an Extended Treatment component. Instead of offering only a few visits to assess problem areas and referring appropriate candidates to other therapists, this service delivery model offers EAP professionals the option of providing extended treatment sessions themselves to employees experiencing most emotional or interpersonal problems. Up to eight visits are available through this EAP model. Only cases requiring extensive treatment (such as medication, structural outpatient substance abuse programs), specialized services, or inpatient stabilization would be referred to outside providers or facilities.

Employee Assistance Programs offering expanded managed care functions, all through one vendor, are of interest to many employers. These EAPs provide easy access to employees, referral to a credentialed, contracted, provider network, and the availability of utilization management specialists.

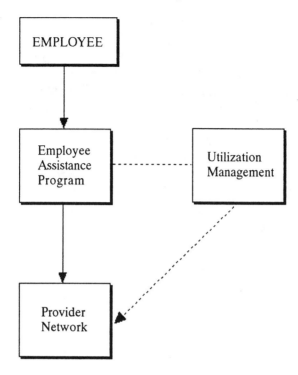

This Extended Treatment version EAP is attractive to employees who can receive this counseling at no out-of-pocket expense. They can continue with their initial counselor avoiding a disruptive referral to a new therapist. They will view this service as another logical step in the evolving process whereby the institution of the "workplace" facilitates access for its valuable employees to diverse employer-sponsored health, educational, and social services once the domain of other institutions in American life.

To the employer, this model offers the flexibility of structuring these important counseling sessions along the lines it desires concerning sites and locations. The counselors provide the therapy work for the employer, in contrast to private practitioners over whose practice orientations employers have much less control. Instead, these counselors will work toward returning the employee to his or her normal level of functioning as soon as possible, having no incentive to "overtreat" or to overutilize costly inpatient resources.

Importantly, employers using this Extended Treatment component EAP will be able to reduce expensive health care benefits, aware that there will be no loss of service availability to employees who will access mental health services through their EAP counselors. Employers who will utilize this model EAP must be careful to ensure adequate levels of staff training, clinical supervision, and psychiatrist involvement so as to avoid shortcomings in client care. Employers should evaluate the treatment outcomes achieved by their staff and closely monitor client satisfaction.

To EAP professionals, this model represents an opportunity to expand their traditional professional role, to the betterment of both the employee and the employer. EAP staff utilizing this model must become skilled in the "brief" or solution-focused therapy techniques.* They must also look to researchers to inform them as to which conditions are most amenable to treatment within the confines of the program and to answer other questions related to client service and treatment outcomes.

Described below are EAP case studies, the latter utilizing an extended treatment component. One involves a large, national employer, the second is a medium-sized company. Both use retooled EAP models featuring managed care functions.

Black and Decker Corporation, headquartered in Towson, Maryland, recently contracted with MCC Companies, a division of CIGNA, to provide a nationwide EAP with an EPO component for ten thousand of its employees. In addition to its customary EAP aspects, a feature to this EAP is its mandatory nature concerning access to mental health and substance abuse benefits. An employee wanting to use these benefits calls a toll free telephone number,

---

*Most courses of therapy in the United States are delivered in a few sessions. Developments in the area of time-sensitive therapies will help counselors achieve even more rapid results. See Pekarik, G. and Wierzbicki, M. "The Relationship Between Clients' Expected and Actual Treatment Duration." *Psychotherapy* Vol. 23, No. 4, 1986. pp. 532-534; Koss, M. P. "Length of psychotherapy for clients seen in private practice." *Journal of Consulting and Clinical Psychology*, Vol. 47, 1979. pp. 210-212; and NIMH, "Provisional data on federally funded community mental health centers, 1978-79." Report prepared by the Survey and Reports Branch, Division of Biometry and Epidemiology, Washington, DC: U.S. Government Printing Office.

accessing an EAP counselor who, after verifying eligibility, assesses the problem or complaint. The employee is then referred to a provider of treatment services that is affiliated with MCC's nationwide network of providers. Or, the employee may receive an appointment at one of the firm's numerous clinics, utilizing an automated, electronic scheduling system. The same system communicates the authorization for services to the clinic. Indemnity insurance claims, paid through a CIGNA claims office, are honored only for services authorized by the EAP, which also provides utilization management and review. In this manner, the employer is able to integrate MMHC and EAP function and interface them with an existing indemnity claims payor, while taking advantage of a managed care network of providers.

Titmus Optical, Inc. is a Petersburg, Virginia-based division of Carl Zeiss, the German manufacturer of optical and scientific instruments. As a self-insured employer, it was particularly concerned with escalating mental health care costs. It contracted with MCC to provide an EAP to its employees that featured an extended treatment benefit. In this arrangement, these Titmus employees are eligible for up to eight therapy visits at no out-of-pocket expense. Since many of the problems that bring employees to counseling settings can be resolved within this limit, employees typically do not need further treatment services. For those that do, Titmus negotiated a discounted fee arrangement with MCC, complete with a copayment structure that incented the employee to utilize MCC therapists, rather than access indemnity insurance benefits. As a self-insured company, Titmus is billed directly by MCC for these clinical services provided beyond the EAP extended treatment benefit. In this manner the employer is able to again combine MMHC and EAP functions, utilizing one vendor for both services, while reducing its mental health care costs through the shared risk and discounted fee arrangement with MCC.

As in the above example, employers and the benefits consultants that advise them are becoming increasingly aware of advances in the development of time-sensitive therapies. (These therapy approaches are variously called Problem-Focused, Solution-Focused, Brief Therapy, etc.) As these approaches rapidly gain more adherents and acceptance in the professional community, employers will look toward EAP counselors to deliver more services themselves, resulting in reduced MH/SA claims and subsequent expense.

IMPLICATIONS FOR EAP PROFESSIONALS

How can clinicians in the EAP field best prepare for an increasingly "managed care" practice environment? First, accept that MMHC is a reality. It is here to stay. It has come about in the last ten years or so due in part to the failure of EAPs to achieve organizational goals desired by employers, now being addressed through MMHC functions.

Second, learn about MMHC systems and technologies; expand your knowledge base. Become able to be a well-informed consultant to employers about MMHC. Don't take an adversarial approach. Become sophisticated enough about MMHC to be able to recognize and delineate quality programs from poor ones.

Third, "retool" your practice skills, if need be. Develop skills in time-sensitive therapy approaches, crisis intervention, and assessment and diagnostic, case management, and utilization management skills.

Fourth, and most importantly, be innovative. If you are presently engaged in EAP work, do not let institutional biases deter you from changing your program's service mixture to fit today's and tomorrow's challenges.

If you are marketing new EAPs, be creative and flexible. Listen to employer's needs. Determine how EAPs may be modified or enhanced to meet needs as well or better than MMHC systems.

If you are a clinician who receives referrals from EAPs, learn about the dynamics that are changing EAP practice. Be able to practice and document efficient, high quality care. Consider developing a "niche" for your practice, based on the needs of EAP referral sources. Look for opportunities in this time of change. (See Table 4-2.)

TABLE 4-2. Traditional EAP Model Contrasted with Enhanced EAPs with MMHC Components

A). **Traditional EAP Model**

Direct Client Services	Indirect Services
a. Self/Supervisor identify client	a. Policy Development
b. EAP staff assess client (1-3 visits)	b. Consultation Statistical Reporting
c. EAP staff refers client for treatment to informal network	c. Training
d. EAP Staff provided follow-up and monitoring of case; coordinates with supervisor as needed	
e. Case Closure	

B). **Enhanced EAP - Model One, A Managed Care EAP with a Network**

Direct Client Services	Indirect Services
a. Self/Supervisor/Others identify client	a. Policy Development
b. EAP staff verify eligibility	b. Consultation/ Statistical Reporting
c. EAP staff assess client	c. Training
d. EAP staff educate client about benefits	d. Awareness Activities

TABLE 4-2. (continued)

e. EAP staff refer to a
   Participating Network Provider
   (formal arrangement with
   provider may include acceptance
   of discounted fees)

f. Benefit Design incents client to
   use network provider. Out-of-
   network providers selection is
   still a covered benefit. Incentives
   to the client to use in-network
   providers may include:
   - lower or no copayment
   - no claim forms to complete
   - richer benefits with in-network
     provider
   - broader selection of providers

g. EAP staff provide follow-up and
   monitoring, coordination with
   supervisor if needed

h. Case closure

C). **Enhanced EAP - Model Two, A Managed Care EAP with an Extended Treatment Component, Plus Network.**

Direct Client Services	Indirect Services
a. Self/Supervisor/Others identify client	a. Policy Development
b. EAP staff verify eligibility	b. Consultation/ Statistical Reporting

c. EAP staff assess client

d. EAP staff educate client
   about benefits

e. EAP Staff Clinicians Provide
   Direct Treatment Services to 8
   visit limit. If the need exists for
   further services after the 8th
   visit, the client is referred into
   the Network.*

f. Benefit Design encourages the
   client to use the EAP clinician,
   i.e. at no cost to the employee as
   these services have been pre-paid
   by the employer.

c. Training

d. Awareness Activities

*   This model is in part based on data indicating that most episodes of
psychotherapy or counseling provided by recognized practitioners in the
United States is of a short-term nature and that short-term counseling is
preferred by most individuals. For example, studies have shown that over
70% of consumers expect therapy to last 10 or less visits, while the modal
number of visits to therapists in the U.S is one. Studies show that close to half
of private practice patients are seen four times or less and nearly 3/4
terminate by the tenth visit. This EAP Model provides counseling services at
no cost to the client, in durations that most consumers seem to want, as well as
the duration that office-based practitioners can provide efficaciously to most
clients. (See: National Institute of Mental Health. (1981). Provisional data
on federally funded community mental health centers, 1978-79. Report
prepared by the Survey and Reports Branch, Division of Biometry and

TABLE 4-2. (continued)

Epidemiology. Washington, DC: U.S. Government Printing Office; Pekarik, G. (1983) Follow-up adjustment of outpatients dropouts. American Journal of Orthopsychiatry, 23, 532-534, and Taube, C.A., Burns, B. J., and Kessler, L. (1984). Patients of psychiatrists and psychologists in office-based practice: 1980. American Psychologist, 39, 1435-1447.)

D). Enhanced EAP - Model Two, A Managed Care EAP with Concurrent Review Functions

<u>Direct Client Services</u>

a. Self/Supervisor/other identify

b. EAP staff verifies eligibility

c. EAP staff assess client

d. All clients must be assessed by EAP staff in order to access benefits

e. EAP staff educated client about benefits

f. EAP staff refer client to in-network provider. This is a formal provider network. (Client may opt. for out-of-network provider with inherent disincentives).

<u>Indirect Services</u>

a. Policy Development

b. Consultation/Statistical Reporting

c. Training

d. Awareness Activities

g. EAP staff authorize treatment -
   forwards authorization to
   provider and claims payment
   function.

h. EAP staff pre-certify admissions
   on 24 hours basis.

i. EAP staff provide concurrent
   review of hospital admissions
   and of outpatient care.

j. Benefit Design encourages the client
   to use the EAP Network Provider.

k. Claims function pays providers based
   on EAP authorization (Out-of-Network
   benefits claims payment may be made
   through this operation as well).

l. EAP staff monitor treatment, provide
   follow-up, coordinate with supervisor,
   if needed.

m. Case closure.

REFERENCES

Beiheh, J. K., & Earle, R. H. (1990). *Successful private practice in the 1990's*. New York: Brunner/Mazel Publishers.

Bennet, N., Blum, T., & Roman, P. (1989, March). EAP salary data: Selected results from a national survey. *ALMACAN*, pp. 34-36.

Bureau of National Affairs, Inc. (1987). *EAP: Benefits, problems, and prospects*. Rockville, MD: Author.

Employee Assistance Professional Association. (1990, October). Standards for employee assistance programs. *EAPA Exchange*, [Special section], pp. B-E.

Hickox, R. F. (1990, August). At McDonnell Douglas . . . EAP does it again. *Employee Benefit News*, p.1, 48-49.

Masi, D. (1990, November). (Personal Communication).

Nye, S. G. (1990). *Employee assistance law answer book*. New York: Panel Publishers.

Smollen, E. (1990, November). Certification update. *Employee Assistance*, pp. 35-36.

Staff. (1989, August). McDonnell Douglas Corporation's EAP produces hard data. ALMACAN, pp. 18-26.

Walker, P. L. (1990, August). EAP education. *Employee Assistance*, pp. 28-30.

Wenzel, L. (1990, July). Let's take credit for being the good case managers that we are. *EAPA Exchange*, p.16.

Wrich, J. T. (1980). *The employee assistance program*. Center City, MN: Hazelden.

Chapter Five

Managed Mental Health Care Systems

In recent years the technologies used in the alternative health care delivery systems described earlier have made their impact on mental health and substance abuse (MH/SA) treatment. Increased sophistication on the part of employers and insurance carriers, spiralling MH/SA benefit costs, better information gathering, and new treatment approaches have created the dynamics which are profoundly changing practice patterns in mental health. The result has been a wide range of evolving mental health and substance abuse treatment delivery systems and benefit designs.

This section will focus on these new managed mental health care systems and technologies that promise to revolutionize professional practice in the 1990s. Before beginning, however, it is useful to consider various MMHC systems in terms of the following qualities and variables:

- *Compensation for Services.* How is the MMHC system's staff compensated?
- *Gatekeeping.* To what extent does the MMHC system assess the need for and direct the patient toward the appropriate type, level, intensity, and duration of care, and type of treatment provider?
- *Consumer Choice.* To what extent does the MMHC system maximize or limit consumer choice of the type and level of care and/or treatment provider? Are a variety of convenient providers and services available?
- *Utilization Management.* To what extent does the MMHC system provide for various utilization management functions?
- *Treatment Provision.* To what extent does the MMHC system provide treatment services through its own staff and clinics

versus managing benefits and services through a network of providers?

- *Cost Savings to Purchaser.* To what extent does the MMHC system obtain cost savings to the employer, HMO, or insurance carrier?
- *Case Management.* To what extent does the MMHC provide for the ongoing monitoring of the clinical care and authorization of reimbursement for the resources allocated to the care?
- *Quality Assurance Oversight.* Who provides their oversight? Is the oversight internally or externally provided? Is the MMHC system regulated or licensed by third parties? Are its staff licensed?

Table 5-1 compares various MMHC systems concerning these qualities.

These characteristics, which have much significance to purchasers of services and to treatment professionals, may have less meaning to the typical consumer of MH/SA treatment services. Often, from the consumer's perspective, freedom of choice in selecting MH/SA treatment resources is the most important quality. Figure 5-1 describes MMHC systems (beginning with unmanaged indemnity insurance as a starting point) for this quality alone.

MMHC FUNDAMENTALS

The fact that there are no standard models of MMHC systems contributes to much of the confusion concerning their operations and objectives. As with any other industry, the more efficient and effective models will survive and proliferate in the marketplace, so the coming years will witness refinement in present-day systems. Rather than attempt to describe all possible permutations of current MMHC systems, this section will focus on the common functions and mechanisms found in most such operations. As we will see, much MMHC technology is derived from HMO and PPO forms.

TABLE 5-1. Comparison of Managed Mental Health Care Systems

	Indemnity* Insurance (unmanaged)	Traditional Employee Assistance Programs	Modified Employee Assistance Programs, with Networks	MMHC Provider Networks	MMHC Exclusive Provider Organizations with Networks	MMHC Exclusive Provider Organizations without Networks
Compensation for Services Delivered	Fee-For-Service with various deductibles	Salaried Employees of Company or Contractors	Salaried Staff, discounted fee-for-service arrangements, etc.	Salaried Staff, discounted fee-for-service arrangements, etc.	Salaried Employees of MMHC System and Fee-For Service with copayments	Salaried Employees of MMHC System
Gatekeeping	None	Limited	Moderate	Moderate	Maximum	Maximum
Consumer Choice	Maximum	Moderate, EAP recommends treatment resources	Moderate, EAP uses Network	Moderate, MMHC uses Network	Limited	None
Utilization Management	None	None	Limited	Moderate	Maximum	Maximum
Treatment Provision	Treatment	No Treatment	Treatment through Network	Treatment Provided	Treatment Provided	Treatment Provided
Estimated Cost Savings to Purchaser of System	None	Limited	Moderate	Moderate	Maximum	Maximum
Case Management	None	Limited	Moderate	Moderate	Maximum	Maximum
Quality Assurance Oversight	Minimal	Minimal	Various Q.A. functioning, internal & external	Various Q.A. functioning, internal & external	Various Q.A. functioning, internal & external	Various Q.A. functioning, internal & external

* As Compared to MMHC's

FIGURE 5-1. MMHC Systems and Consumer Choice of Treatment and Treatment Provider

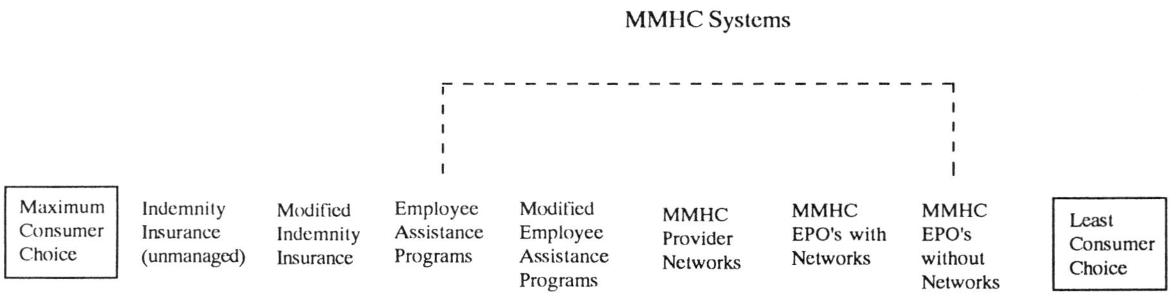

MMHC Systems

| Maximum Consumer Choice | Indemnity Insurance (unmanaged) | Modified Indemnity Insurance | Employee Assistance Programs | Modified Employee Assistance Programs | MMHC Provider Networks | MMHC EPO's with Networks | MMHC EPO's without Networks | Least Consumer Choice |

Values and Beliefs Associated with MMHC

All industries reflect certain values in their day-to-day operations. This is true in the MMHC field as well. Their values impact both the clinical and administrative aspects of their activities. MMHC values are probably shared by a large proportion of practitioners and administrators today. Others view MMHC's philosophies as an unpalatable departure from traditional themes long found in the health care field.

MMHC bases much of its structure on the belief that most people can "get better" (recover, overcome their presenting problem, find a solution, etc.) and that they want to improve as quickly as possible. As a result, those in the MMHC field view themselves as advocates for clients since they see MMHC as an avenue to help consumers achieve this goal of rapid change and improvement. Also, MMHC systems tend to focus on clinical technologies that help people achieve this goal of returning to their normal status or highest level of functioning as quickly as possible. Related to this belief is the notion that most consumers want help with specific, not global, problems and that treatment can be intermittent since specific problems needing professional attention may come and go over the course of a lifetime. Clinicians who hold this belief view themselves, in effect, as providing needed "tune ups," not full engine overhauls.

A belief in the importance of efficiency is inherent in MMHC. While critics have said that MMHC's quest for efficiency sometimes overlooks client care, clinicians in these systems believe that a lack of efficiency in many aspects of traditional mental health delivery systems escalates costs to consumers unnecessarily. When taken to the last degree, this escalation endangers mental health and substance abuse treatment benefits for many Americans.

Another belief common to MMHC is that treatment is best delivered in the least restrictive and most normal setting possible. Outpatient treatment is stressed. MMHC clinicians believe that most consumers prefer this orientation and desire treatment that is the least invasive and least disruptive possible. Related to this is the belief that hospital resources for MMHC clients are needed for stabilization of acute crisis, and that the primary treatment should be provided on an outpatient basis when the client's condition permits. MMHC clinicians point out that while this belief is prevalent in other health care fields mental health practitioners and institutions have been slow to embrace the idea.

Unlike some indemnity insurance plans which limit reimbursable provider status to one or two professions, many MMHC managers believe a range of providers is desirable. They believe this gives their clients greater choice, better access in some areas, and increased treatment options. This value is frequently operationalized through staffs and provider networks that feature not only psychiatrists and psychologists, but also clinical social workers, professional counselors, marriage and family therapists, clinical nurse specialists, and substance abuse counselors.

MMHC stresses the belief that adequate clinical case management improves the continuity of care. These systems designate a "case manager" who has responsibility for the overall coordination (both clinical and financial aspects) of the client's care throughout a treatment episode. Clinicians in MMHC believe this case management function greatly assists the client in transversing various treatment pitfalls and reduces the likelihood of wasting treatment resources through ineffectiveness, inefficiency, or duplication.

While focusing on such "micro" management of care and resources, MMHC systems also value the "macro" management of the resources needed to provide care for large populations of patients, a different perspective than that normally taken in everyday practice. They attempt to achieve economies of scale, obtain favorable pricing and charge arrangements, and in other ways manage resources so as to obtain optimum, if not maximum, care for each member.

Finally, MMHC's philosophy is that much care delivered to consumers today is unnecessary; much other care is ineffective. More care does not necessarily mean better care. MMHC views these factors as weighing heavily in the escalating costs of mental health and substance abuse care. It operates with the belief that these escalating costs, unless checked, will force employers to reduce or eliminate MH/SA benefits from their health care benefit plans entirely. They believe that MMHC, with its emphasis on accountability and structure, can ensure necessary and cost-effective care for its members. The rapid growth of MMHC in recent years has been an endorsement of this belief by the ultimate major purchasers of mental health care: employers.

ELEMENTS OF MMHC SYSTEMS

Managed Mental Health Care systems have four core elements and a range of secondary elements. The components can be delivered to HMO or Employer customers either by specialty, MMHC firms or by Employee Assistance Program (EAP) firms. Core elements include:

- Gatekeeping
- Provider Network Development
- Utilization Management*
- Clinical Case Management

Secondary elements or functions of these systems include:

- Benefits Design or Re-design
- Eligibility Verification
- Benefits Interpretation
- Emergency Intervention and Access
- Evaluation
- Employee Assistance Functions (training, awareness and education activities)
- Quality Assurance
- Claims Processing and Adjudication

(See Figures 5-2, 5-3, and 5-4.)

This chapter explores how the functions of these various aspects of MMHC systems work, how patients are served, and how providers are utilized. MMHC is a growth industry and an emerging field of practice for mental health clinicians and administrators. The reader will find that often MMHC systems parallel the HMO models described in Chapter Two, yet many variations exist. No

---

*Discussed in Chapter Six

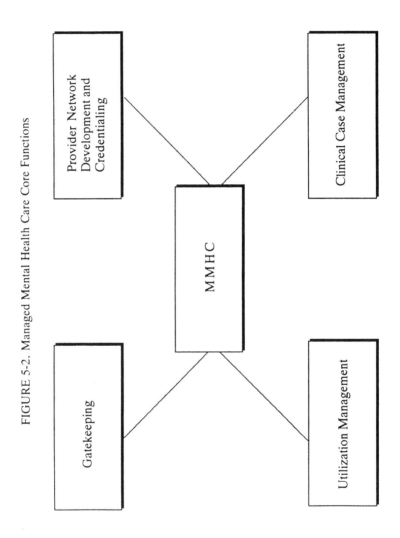

FIGURE 5-2. Managed Mental Health Care Core Functions

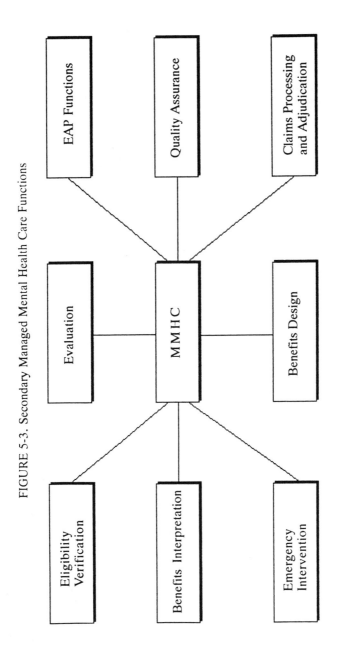

FIGURE 5-3. Secondary Managed Mental Health Care Functions

FIGURE 5-4. MMHC Client Flow Chart

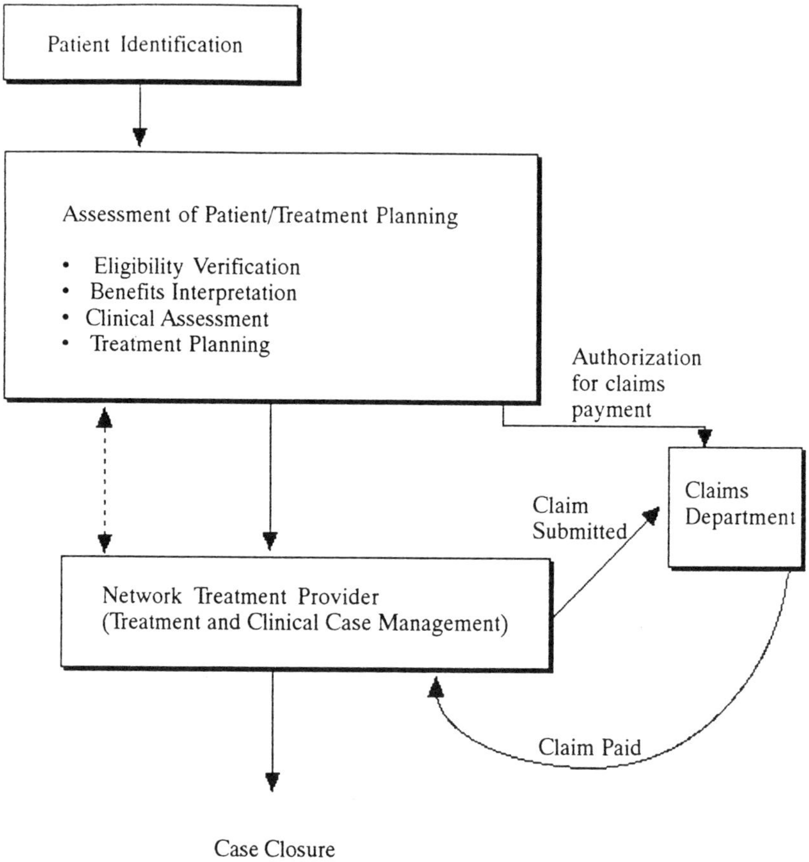

```
┌─────────────────────────────┐
│  Patient Identification      │
└─────────────────────────────┘
              │
              ▼
┌─────────────────────────────────────────────┐
│  Assessment of Patient/Treatment Planning    │
│                                               │
│   •  Eligibility Verification                 │
│   •  Benefits Interpretation                  │
│   •  Clinical Assessment                      │
│   •  Treatment Planning                       │
└─────────────────────────────────────────────┘
```

Authorization
for claims
payment

Claim
Submitted

Claims
Department

Network Treatment Provider
(Treatment and Clinical Case Management)

Claim Paid

Case Closure

one "model" prevails. A familiarity with these core functions provides a basis for understanding the mechanics of this industry.

Gatekeeping

In medical HMOs the Primary Care Physician (PCP) serves as the gatekeeper to all of the system's services such as specialty care, testing, or inpatient treatment. MMHC clinicians serve this gatekeeping function concerning mental health and substance abuse services.

The gatekeeper's objectives are twofold: assessment and treatment planning. First, the client's presenting problem is assessed and a diagnostic impression is reached. Second, the type, level, and intensity of treatment, and the provider type are matched to the presenting problem. This treatment plan and designated provider or facility are then authorized for coverage through the client's benefit plan. This task requires substantial skill, experience, and expertise. A thorough knowledge of available community resources is also invaluable. These clinical decisions are often made in multidisciplinary team meetings. The input from clinicians of different professional training and backgrounds strengthens these decisions.

If conducted improperly, this gatekeeping function can have negative consequences for both the client and the MMHC organization. For example, if, due to a diagnostic error, the recommended treatment is not the most effective one available, or if it is not delivered as intensively as needed, the client may not improve. The client may present again at a later time in a deteriorated condition, requiring more intensive (and expensive) care. The result is that the client has not been well served toward his or her goal of improvement, while the MMHC firm has incurred more costs than would have been necessary had care been effective initially.

This gatekeeping function may be provided by a MMHC firm's employees or by contracted providers. It is usually conducted by nonphysician clinicians in consultation with a psychiatrist. A more intensive assessment utilizing medical personnel is frequently provided to substance abuse or other clients presenting with medical complications. In some HMO systems, a referral to the MMHC staff for assessment and treatment occurs only after a PCP has assessed the client, ruling out purely medical etiologies.

Gatekeeping is a key aspect of MMHC systems and helps to reduce unnecessary and costly care. Its greatest impact concerns unnecessary hospital care, the most costly segment of mental health and substance abuse treatment. The gatekeeping function requires, in effect, clinical assessment before hospitalization. This function (along with Pre-Admission Certification, discussed later) eliminates or reduces the consumer's choice of and ability to select costly inpatient treatment modalities, without assessment by nonhospital affiliated clinicians.*

Provider Networks

After assessment and treatment planning, MMHC clients are directed toward providers who are affiliated with the MMHC firm. This is said to be the MMHC firm's provider network. Care is then authorized for reimbursement to the providers who are members of the network. Provider network members are recruited, or selected for inclusion, based on several factors. These include clinical skills and services, geographical considerations, cost-effective practice patterns, congruent values with MMHC systems, and willingness to comply with utilization review processes. Providers are "credentialed" by the MMHC firm as a quality assurance measure. This process may entail the submission by the provider of documentation of a professional license, educational background, DEA registration (where appropriate), adequate malpractice insurance coverage, the absence of misconduct or ethical violations, and the adequacy of emergency access for referred clients. MMHC groups confirm such documentation with licensure boards and other entities when appropriate. Credentials of providers are periodically reviewed and updated. MMHC staff usually interview potential providers to assess clinical skills and to orient them to the system.

Providers sign agreements with MMHC firms that contain various stipulations about service and reimbursement arrangements. A schedule of allowable fee maximums is agreed upon for the services the provider will render to MMHC clients. Like HMO-PCP agreements, these arrangements prohibit the provider from billing the client inappropriately, prescribe mechanisms for the resolution of disputes, discuss the confidentiality of client information, and indicate what type of services the provider will deliver. Examples of provider credentialing materials and a sample provider agreement are found in Appendix A.

MMHC firms further their goals of providing cost-effective,

---

*This gatekeeping function, especially vis-à-vis hospitalization, is also exemplified by many Community Mental Health Centers (CMHCs).

quality care through the utilization of provider networks. Cost savings are achieved through recruiting effective and efficient service providers, while obtaining a discounted fee arrangement (a reduction of 15% or more of usual charges is often obtained). At the same time their credentialing and screening process ensures that quality services will be offered to their clients.

To providers, affiliation has some drawbacks and several advantages. An obvious drawback is the discounted fee requested by the MMHC entity. In addition, the credentialing and utilization review processes may present additional paperwork and be time consuming tasks. (Obviously those providers or facilities who are not philosophically attuned to MMHC or whose treatment preferences are not compatible with MMHC's authorization patterns will find network affiliation difficult or problematic.) However, membership in one or more MMHC networks can ensure a steady source of referrals. In communities with an overabundance of facilities or individual providers, such an affiliation may be crucial and may be an important means of developing a successful practice (see Chapter Eight for more discussion of this issue).

Networks may be as large or as small as the MMHC requires in order to serve its members. Networks may include only such facilities as hospitals or detoxification centers, or they may include only individual outpatient practitioners; often they include both. In determining the size and composition of their networks, MMHCs consider factors such as their member population's utilization of services history (which can be analyzed by examining past claim submission data), the geographical distribution of members, the quality of service delivery and practice patterns of the community of providers, and customer input concerning the provider network. A large consideration on the part of MMHC is the cost-effectiveness of a provider network applicant's practice. Firms have successfully resisted efforts by groups of providers for automatic inclusion in such networks. Obviously, if all providers or all hospitals in a given community were network members, any cost-effective practice on the part of some would be offset by the lack of such practice on the part of others, thus negating an important MMHC objective.

The way in which networks are utilized varies. In some arrangements, an MMHC client is assessed by a staff clinician of the firm.

Treatment is then authorized to be conducted at the office of a network provider. In other arrangements, the client may seek assessment with any MMHC network provider. The provider then communicates the assessment information to the MMHC staff, who authorize further care with the provider. Still other arrangements include specially designated network providers who provide assessment only, while treatment services are offered through other providers. Although this procedure may inconvenience the client (who must see both an assessment clinician and a treatment clinician), it removes any incentive for the assessor to recommend treatment that would benefit the assessor's practice. By modifying these assessment and treatment provision arrangements, MMHC firms may share gatekeeping responsibilities with network providers.

The proportion of treatment services delivered by the network versus the MMHC staff may vary as well. In some instances the MMHC firm functions only as a developer and manager of a MH/SA preferred provider organization, providing little or no treatment services.

For example, the ACME FLANGE Company is a large self-insured employer with factory operations in three cities and a small sales force scattered about the nation. ACME's benefit manager, working with his benefit consultant, decides that ACME will take steps to control the cost of its MH/SA claims, after it is realized that these claims are inordinately costly in relation to all health care claims submitted by ACME's employees. One strategy ACME will use, they decide, is to employ a MMHC firm to develop and administer a network of cost-effective providers and facilities for their employees in various locations. They select a firm that already has networks of providers in two of the three cities and most of the locations of their sales force. The firm is quickly able to recruit and credential a network in the third city. ACME wishes its employees to have immediate access to these providers, so the gatekeeping function is also delegated to the respective provider selected by the employee, and is essentially deemphasized. ACME "purchases" the MMHC's network, i.e., its ability to develop and administer a network of cost-effective service providers. The firm receives an administrative fee from ACME. Its providers receive more referrals. ACME receives quality services for its employees while enjoying the cost savings associated with their discounted fees and cost-effective practice patterns. In this example ACME continues to be at risk financially for the cost of services and continues to utilize a third party administrator (TPA) to process and pay claims.

In other scenarios, an MMHC firm might utilize network providers minimally. MMHC entities may utilize their own staff to provide most services. When an MMHC firm assumes the risk for the services of HMO members, it may wish to control costs by having a limited provider network and instead employ staff to provide most of the services its members require. It becomes the exclusive provider network for MH/SA care to the HMO's members. In this scenario, the MMHC firm might utilize a network only for specialized services or inpatient care. To a large extent, the MMHC firm has internalized its network, employing practitioners directly. These configurations have many of the advantages and disadvantages of administration that are inherent to staff model medical/surgical HMOs.

How the MMHC firm utilizes its network may also change with time as its relationship to its accounts (customers) changes. Returning to the ACME FLANGE Company example, after one year's experience with the arrangement described, ACME reevaluates its benefits for mental health and substance abuse treatment in light of continuing cost increases in its health care claims and its sagging profits. In reviewing the MMHC network's performance, it finds that most of its employees are using its members as opposed to other providers. However, it finds that employees are often selecting the most costly providers for services that could be as effectively delivered by other professionals.

In view of this development, ACME asks the MMHC to increase its gatekeeping function, focusing on matching the treatment need with the least costly provider who can appropriately deliver necessary services. The MMHC firm responds by designating its staff clinicians in one city and selected network assessment providers in the other locations to serve as gatekeepers to the system. The gatekeepers are able to direct referrals to network providers on a more cost-effective basis, better matching the level of treatment need with level of provider. (In actual operation this might mean that psychologists, licensed clinical social workers, professional counselors, or marriage and family therapists would be authorized to perform more counseling services, while psychiatrists in the network would be authorized for therapy services that only they are skilled in and qualified to provide.)

Through the MMHC firm's services, ACME is able to gain more control of its costs at the expense of some choice on the part of its employees. ACME's management had exercised this choice in advance, by purchasing this gatekeeping function through the MMHC firm.

Clinical Case Management

This term refers to the assortment of activities concerning the coordination and monitoring of client services throughout the treatment episode. The development of this function in MMHC systems parallels that of the PCP who is medical case manager in HMOs. It also reflects the belief on the part of MMHCs that treatment resources are misused in the absence of clinical oversight. This function in MMHC arrangements is the key to the management of care.

Important aspects of the clinical case manager function include:

- coordination of care with treatment providers
- coordination of care with PCPs and other medical services
- referral to available community resources for additional services not included in the client's benefits (examples include self-help or support group referrals)
- benefit interpretation

The clinical case manager may be the treatment provider (as in the case of staff model operations) or may be the MMHC staff member who consults with the treatment provider and performs concurrent review functions. (See Chapter Six for a discussion of this and other utilization review functions in MMHC systems.) In either situation, the clinical case manager is the point of interface between the client and available treatment resources. (See Table 5-2.)

TABLE 5-2. Steps in the MMHC Clinical Case Management Process

Case Identification
- Self-initiated
- Family, physician, employer initiated

Assessment of Patient
- Benefit eligibility determination
- Benefits interpretation
- Clinical assessment
- Diagnosis established

Treatment Plan Development
- Type of treatment determined
- Setting for treatment determined
- Intensity of treatment determined
- Duration of treatment estimated
- Providers of treatment determined
- Patient (and family/employers) agrees to treatment plan

Treatment Plan Implementation/Monitoring
- Arrangements made with provider for service delivery
- Transfer of patient coordinated
- Reimbursement arrangements coordinated
- Authorization written for claims payment
- Treatment progress monitored, treatment plan modified as needed

Case Closure

Additional Functions

Several additional functions are available through MMHC firms. Some may be viewed as add-ons to essential components. Essential components include eligibility verification and benefits interpretation. These are straightforward tasks. When a client accesses services, his name is verified as an active, eligible member of the benefit or group health plan. Rosters of members are kept current according to changes in employee groups or health care plan membership. This is a clerical function, while interpretation of benefits is an important clinical function involving the case manager. In each case benefits must be interpreted as they pertain to the client's assessment. Excluded conditions and benefit limitations must be considered in this task. MMHC must be judicious concerning benefit interpretation, providing only the services previously contracted for with the customer. A common abuse of benefit interpretation can occur in the unmanaged practice environment when the clinician interprets benefits to cover services he or she is accustomed to providing, such as long-term psychotherapy aimed at characterological change or marriage counseling even though neither is actually a covered benefit.

Another essential aspect of MMHC is emergency intervention. MMHC administrators realize that psychiatric crises occur at all hours, so their systems must be organized so as to offer accessible crisis counseling at all times. Prompt intervention also can diffuse many crises and thereby prevent a costly hospitalization.

Benefits design consultation is also offered by MMHC entities. In the example of ACME, benefits were changed so as to encourage the utilization of outpatient care and the designated provider network. Prior to the introduction of managed care, ACME's benefits paid 100% of the employee's inpatient claims, while only paying 50% of outpatient claims. ACME's MMHC firm recommended changes resulting in a structure featuring employee cost-sharing, and incenting the employee to use ACME's network. Table 5-3 shows how ACME's new benefit design works, providing coverage for employees who use the network providers as well as for those who do not.

Some large MMHC entities may also process, adjudicate, and pay claims as well as provide evaluation or outcome studies about treatment. Some firms regularly survey their clients concerning clinical services provided by their staff or network providers and facilities, utilizing this data in management decision making.

MMHC firms also have various quality assurance features, some of which may interface with those of their HMO customers. These include peer reviews, random chart audits, examination or audits of readmissions to hospitals within a prescribed period (thirty days for example), examination or audits of reapplications for outpatient care, credentialing and updating of provider credentials, and compliance with state regulatory agencies. Many MMHC firms, especially those who provide direct treatment services, may be licensed and regulated for mental health and substance abuse services by state regulatory entities. Licensure of individual practitioners em-

TABLE 5-3. ACME Benefits

In-Network Benefits   Out - of Network Benefits

Mental Health

Outpatient

up to 20 visits $10 copayment (individual Tx)   70% coverage
per year $ 5 copayment (group Tx)   of charges after
                                                        meeting $250
                                                         deductible

Inpatient

up to 30 days   20% copayment   70% coverage of
per year; 2-1   of charges after
conversion to   meeting $500
partial hospitalization days   deductible

Substance Abuse

Outpatient

up to 20 visits $ 5 copayment (group TX)   70% coverage
per year; $ 10 copayment (individual TX)   of charges after
unlimited group   meeting $250
treatment   deductible

Inpatient

up to 30 days   20% copayment   70% coverage of
per year; 2-1   of charges after
conversion to   meeting $500
partial hospitalization days   deductible

ployed directly by the MMHC firm is yet another level of quality assurance.

Finally, with convergence of MMHC and EAP functions, many firms are able to offer the supervisory training, employee education and other components of traditional EAPs, rounding out the constellation of services available to employer accounts.

Internal Organization and Staffing Patterns

MMHC systems that provide assessment and treatment services directly to clients (as opposed to those that only manage benefits) are often clinically organized to resemble other large counseling concerns, such as group practices, private clinics, or community mental health centers. Their internal operations tend to be focused on the provision of services to acute clients and on helping all clients improve on a timely basis. Many offer intensive outpatient substance abuse programs, partial hospitalization, crisis intervention teams, and ambulatory detoxification. Group therapy programs are used as well.

Some administrative organizational structures may be centralized while others are retained on local levels. For example, a large MMHC company may have one centralized customer service department, responding to member inquiries or provider questions, while each local office may carry out some customer service functions. Management information systems, tracking service utilization data and generating summary reports may be best done on a centralized basis, as may claims processing.

Staff positions within these systems parallel those in other counseling settings. Administrative titles include "Executive Director" or "Network Manager." Psychiatrists in such systems hold positions such as "Medical Director" or "Consultant." They provide direct services and supervision of clinical and utilization review processes. Clinical directors are often senior clinicians with responsibility for overall staff services and training. MMHC entities may also have staff positions relating to the coordination of quality assurance activities and substance abuse treatment services.

In a 1988 report reporting concerning 1986 surveys of HMOs, Shadle and Christianson found wide variation in the ratio of MMHC staff to members (commonly expressed as a Full Time Equivalent (FTE) per ten thousand-member ratio). These variations are due in large part to the assortment of MMHC arrangements and benefit structures. Given this, a range of one to two FTEs per ten thousand members for nonphysician staff is common in the industry.

What types of mental health clinicians are best suited for the growing employment opportunities in MMHC? First, a great deal of clinical skill and experience is required of clinicians in these challenging systems. Clinicians must be licensed or certified for independent practice and have a thorough knowledge of current clinical practices. Especially important is a familiarity with brief, solution-focused treatment techniques. (See Chapter Eight.)

Some MMHC managers view clinical values as equally important in these settings. "Clinicians from all mental health fields can work well in managed care settings if their values are congruent with managed care practice," says Dr. John Bistline, chairman of the American Mental Health Counselor's Association's Special Interest Network on Managed Care (Personal communication, 1990). Bistline, a supervisor in MMHC systems for five years, believes that MMHC staff who are interested in seeing their clients change quickly, while utilizing the least invasive treatment interventions appropriate, are most successful in these settings.

"The recruitment of staff for MMHC practice is challenging especially concerning psychiatrists," according to Demetrios Julius, MD, a consultant to MCC Companies and to Masi Research Associates, an EAP evaluation firm. Julius, who has been involved in managed health care since the 1970s, advises that a special combination of skills and interests is required.

> First, the psychiatrist must have excellent clinical skills and be abreast of current treatment methodologies and research issues. He must be interested in working as part of a multidisciplinary team. Familiarity with the strengths and limitations of other mental health professionals is important as is the case with other community-oriented psychiatry settings. He also must be philosophically attuned to managed care values, as well as aware of emerging managed care technologies. Finally, the psychiatrist must be comfortable with the evaluative

and peer review nature inherent to these settings. Individuals who combine all these characteristics find managed mental health care to be a good fit and a challenging opportunity. (Personal communication, 1990)

KEY ADMINISTRATIVE ASPECTS OF MMHC SYSTEMS

MMHC firms are constructed in a variety of configurations. A description of all the types is beyond the scope of this book, but certain elements, embodied in almost all such organizations, are relevant to this context. Therefore, this chapter will focus on these aspects:

- Contracts between MMHC firms and their customers
- How MMHC firms are financed
- How MMHC firms measure and use service utilization data

Bear in mind that some MMHC entities also pay claims, develop and administer provider networks only, or provide only employee assistance programming. Also EAPs are increasingly making transitions into MMHC functions. These issues are addressed elsewhere within this book.

This chapter will enable the reader to understand the essentials and speak the language of MMHC utilization data, which measures clinical services in nontraditional ways. We will also explore how utilization projections or estimates, along with the type of services the MMHC is contracted to provide or purchase, derives what it charges to its customers (HMOs or employers). We will examine the pitfalls of this "capitation" funding system which has sometimes resulted in the failure of MMHC organizations, with resultant disruption in patient services and providers' practices.

MMHC Contracts: Key Components

MMHC firms contract with HMOs, insurance carriers, employers, groups of employers, or unions. Like other businesses, these firms are bound by the terms of their agreements; they deliver no more or no fewer services than specified in their agreement. Like any other business they attempt to deliver their services and make a profit. Given the enormous growth of managed care in recent years, these firms have generally been able to do so, while reducing or slowing the cost for MH/SA claims to their customers. Both the firms and their customers relate this accomplishment to MMHC's ability to reduce the use of unnecessary, inefficient, or ineffective care while achieving acceptable levels of customer satisfaction.

Service Standards

Contracts between the MMHC firm and the customer have several important specifications that influence the nature of the service delivery systems. For example, the contract may specify the following various service standards which affect the ultimate configuration of the MMHC operation.

Access Parameters. MMHC contracts specify that initial assessment and diagnostic services will be available to all members. These include provisions for emergency services to clients, twenty-four-hour availability of staff, the availability of routine initial assessments, and geographic service issues such as a standard for reasonable client drive time to a clinic or provider.

Provider Parameters. The customer may specify in the contract how the provider credentialing process will be implemented and monitored, what types of providers may be credentialed, etc.

Quality Assurance Parameters. The customer may specify various functions related to quality oversight including peer review, clinical chart audits, complaint and grievance policies, and appeal procedures.

Utilization Data Reporting. This includes provisions for the type and timing of statistical reports. For example, an HMO which employs a MMHC firm to manage its member's MH/SA benefits might specify that the firm will report utilization of services data, i.e., units of services delivered by employer account. In this way the HMO can monitor, account by account, the total amount of both medical and mental health services delivered to each of its employer groups.

Out-of-Service-Area Emergencies. The MMHC firm and the customer specify how they will manage the care of a member or employee who has a need for treatment while traveling or working outside the normal service area. The financial obligation for the care is also specified.

Benefit Descriptions and Limits. A maximum number of therapy visits and hospital days available are specified. Benefit limits may be described in dollar maximum per year. Benefits may also be limited on a "per lifetime" basis. (Table 5-4 gives an example of typical benefit limits). Benefit descriptions in MMHC contracts

TABLE 5-4. Benefit Description and Limits

MENTAL HEALTH

Outpatient Therapy	20 visits per calendar year
Partial Hospitalization	2 - 1 equivalency to inpatient day maximum
Inpatient Hospitalization	30 days per calendar year

SUBSTANCE ABUSE

Outpatient Therapy	50 visits per year, limited to structured treatment program
Partial Hospitalization	2 -1 equivalency to inpatient day maximum
Inpatient Hospitalization	30 days per calendar year, limited to 60 days per lifetime

specify that only medically necessary services and/or preauthorized services only are covered under the plan or system. Protocols for the coverage of emergency presentations or admissions may also be described.

Copayment or Coinsurance Levels. Copayments by the client are an important contractual provision for MMHC systems. Copayments are widely perceived as a means of cost-sharing and of deterring inappropriate utilization of specialist's services. For example, a HMO may establish a copayment for basic health care (Primary Care Physician visits) at a level of $5 per visit. However, a specialist copayment to the MMHC staff or providers might be $10 or $25 per visit.

Disenrollment Policies. Contracts provide for a process by which a member may be expelled from the MMHC system. Examples include members who refuse to pay necessary copayments, who refuse reasonable treatment plans, or who are abusive to the staff or network providers.

Exclusions

A key aspect of the contract by which MMHC firms operate concerns "exclusions." These are services that the customer has not purchased from the MMHC entity. They are not a "covered benefit" under the health care schema.

Court-Ordered Treatment. Provisions specify that simply because treatment, or treatment with a particular individual or institutional provider, is ordered by a court it will not necessarily be covered by the MMHC system for reimbursement purposes. MMHC systems may cover such treatment if it is assessed by the system as being necessary. A common occurrence in this area involves a court which, in effect, sentences a member to thirty days in a hospital for treatment for a substance abuse related offense. The hospitalization would not be covered by the MMHC firm unless it assessed the hospital care, and its length, as the necessary level of treatment for the client.

Treatment for Disorders Not Shown to Be Amenable to Short-Term Interventions. Since a philosophy of MMHC firms is that treatment should be directed at returning the client to his normal level of functioning, their contracts use this clause to exclude the long-term therapy that may, or may not, be successful at altering basic personality or characterological features. MMHC firms usually serve this population with crisis intervention and other services aimed at stabilization only, not characterological change. This exclusion operates in cases of stable personality disordered clients not in an acute crisis at or near their normal level of functioning. Services for this population would include crisis intervention and stabilization, but not the extensive long-term therapy sometimes provided to this client population.

Experimental Therapies. Provisions are made for the exclusion of untried or unproven treatments (as determined by the HMO's, insurance carrier's, or MMHC firm's medical directors or reviewers.) Examples may include vitamin or nutritional therapies, experimental drug therapies, etc.

Treatment for Disorders Classified on V Code Diagnoses in the DSM-III-R. Marital therapy is usually excluded through this clause.

Table 5-5 summarizes the key features of MMHC contracts that impact clinical services.

TABLE 5-5. MMHC Contracts: Key Components

Service Standards
- Access Parameters
- Provider Parameters
- Quality Assurance Parameters
- Utilization Data Reporting
- Out-Of-Service-Area Emergencies
- Benefit Descriptions and Limits
- Copayment Or Coinsurance Levels
- Disenrollment Policies

Exclusions
- Court-Ordered Treatment
- Treatment for Disorders Not Shown to Be Amenable to Short-Term Interventions
- Experimental Therapies
- Treatment for Disorders Classified on V Code Diagnoses in the DSM-III-R

Financing

MMHC systems can be funded in several ways. The most common funding mechanism, capitation, will be discussed here as it applies to an HMO population. Employers may also purchase MMHC services through capitation arrangements.

Just as HMO members pay a fixed fee and in turn receive all their health care services, MMHC firms are often funded through a similar mechanism. Arriving at this "price" for a contract is a vitally important process.

The MMHC group will carefully study the demographics and utilization of services history of any prospective group of members (HMO members, employee population, etc.). Large MMHC firms employ specialists in this process. An MMHC organization will carefully study the benefit schedule that the prospective customer desires, as well as proposed exclusions to the benefit plan. It also will evaluate its own history of managing such benefits.

Other factors important in formulating a capitation figure include local cost considerations, such as hospital costs; provider availability, quality, and familiarity with managed care systems; and other market-specific factors.

A capitation rate* or cap. rate will then be proposed and negotiated between the MMHC firm and its customer. This number, multiplied by the current number of members, will be paid to the MMHC firm each month. From this revenue, plus possible copayment revenue, the MMHC firm must finance all aspects of its operation.

In this scenario, the MMHC firm is then fully at risk for the cost of all clinical services needed by its members. The financial risk for mental health care has been transferred from the HMO or self-insured employer to the MMHC entity. Figures 5-5 and Table 5-6

---

*Capitation is paid each month and is based on the number of actual enrollees in the plan that month. Since plan membership varies from month to month, the capitation revenue may vary correspondingly. Capitation is said to be a "per member, per month" (pm pm) figure.

FIGURE 5-5. Capitation

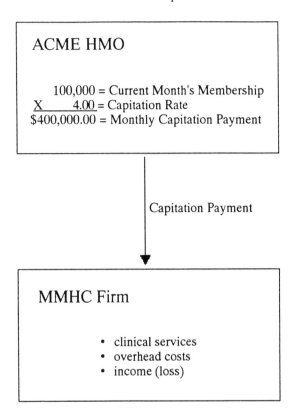

show examples of how capitation funds an MMHC system in which the respective parties have agreed upon a $4 pm pm.*

This type of funding system is found in a modified form in Employee Assistant Program (EAP) services. EAPs traditionally have not been financially at risk for all clinical services, and therefore their charges have been considerably less than MMHC groups. As EAPs evolve towards providing more MMHC functions, this will

---

*Actual capitation rates vary widely depending on the above factors. A range of $1.00 to $5.00 pm pm is common. This contrasts with MMHC's forerunner, Employee Assistance Programs which are often priced at $1.25 to $2.50 per employee, per month (pe pm).

TABLE 5-6. Capitation Funding of MMHC Systems

Revenue:	$4000,000	(Current month's membership X Capitation rate or 100,000 X $4.00)
Cost of Services:	$300,000	(75% of Revenues)
General and Administrative Expenses:	$60,000	(15% of Revenues)
Income:	$40,000	(10% of Revenues)

change. (See Chapter Four for a discussion of EAPs and how they may change in the future as a response to MMHC systems.)

In providing their products, EAPs are typically funded on a "per employee, per year" (pe py) basis. For example, to serve an employer account of one thousand employees the EAP firm might charge $15 pe py or $15,000 annually.

These capitated funding arrangements offer a simplified payment system, but one that is also filled with pitfalls, especially for MMHC groups and their members. Many such organizations, particularly smaller ones or poorly managed ones, have learned this painful lesson and have failed. There are several ways this can occur. Some common scenarios follow.

Apple MMHC contracts with Bob's HMO (an IPA model), which has a membership of fifty thousand, at a cap. rate of $4 pm pm, or $200,000 per month. Administrative and clinical staff are hired, a network of providers is established, and two offices are leased, since the HMO serves a widely dispersed membership. Apple plans to assess all new clients, then refer them for treatment services into its newly recruited provider network. One provider group, confident of securing all of Apple's substance abuse clients, expands its practice, leasing new office space and hiring an additional clinician.

For six months all goes well for Apple. Its assessment function guides their members to the appropriate level of care and into their network of cost-effective practitioners. Apple is profitable, its members receive good care, and its providers receive a steady flow of referrals. Then, totally unrelated to Apple MMHC's services, the HMO loses two important physician groups from its medical panel. Several large employer accounts choose not to renew their business with the HMO, since its primary medical care panel of physicians is no longer as attractive to their employees as it once was. The HMO looses 40% of its membership in a period of a few months. Apple's monthly capitation check shrinks correspondingly. No business can absorb such a dramatic loss of revenue without parallel cutbacks and layoffs. Apple mismanages the necessary transition and is not able to reduce its overhead costs quickly enough. Providers are alienated when referral streams slow down. Apple becomes absorbed with its internal cost of operation issues with resulting poor claims payment and member service problems. The business eventually fails. Client care is disrupted as the HMO must secure a new MMHC organization. Providers, especially the ones that expanded their practices to accommodate Apple's referrals, are further alienated as their businesses feel the ripple effect of the failure. The HMO is further damaged in the marketplace by this setback to its MMHC firm.

This scenario represents the fact that MMHC firms are dependent on a stable HMO population. Changes in the population must be adjusted to quickly and efficiently, with minimal disruption to core MMHC functions. In this way the health of a MMHC firm is connected to the overall well-being of the HMO customer.

Another example demonstrates how too small a revenue base can affect MMHC organizations. In this case, Drs. Smith and Jones decide to pursue a capitated arrangement for Smalltime HMO's mental health needs. Smalltime is actually part of a "big time" insurance carrier, but is in a weak position in Smith and Jones' market. Smalltime has only fifteen thousand members, but their parent insurance company is committed to their presence in this market. Drs. Smith and Jones are confident of success as they launch into the new field of managed care!

Contract in hand, they go about restructuring their practice. They decide they will serve as an exclusive provider organization to Smalltime's members. They hope their new service, a partial hospitalization program, will help them avoid costly inpatient hospitalizations. Also, they hope their managed care contract, with its monthly "cap. check," will finance the partial hospitalization service which they market in the community, generating more revenue. Smalltime will be their cash cow!

Smith and Jones soon fail. An autopsy reveals their MMHC practice underestimated the actual need for inpatient hospitalization and overestimated their partial hospitalization program's ability to circumvent inpatient admissions. Further, the relatively small size of their membership made it difficult for them to negotiate discounted charges from their hospital network. They could not provide the volume of hospital days needed to encourage the hospital administrators to discount their usual rates. Therefore, both the number of hospital days used by their members as well as the cost per day of hospitalization exceeded their estimates. Finally, the doctors were unable to effectively market their partial hospitalization to the community to supplement their contractual revenues.

Had Drs. Smith and Jones anticipated these problems, they would have negotiated a larger cap. rate which would have enabled them to weather the difficult early phase of establishing their managed care practice. They may have been able to reduce the rate charged to Smalltime HMO, the next year, or reduce the expected increase of the rate over subsequent years, once they became accustomed to "managing" the relatively small membership. As with HMOs, MMHC firms often experience higher utilization of hospital beds during the start-up phase of operation. Utilization of bed days on this scenario would probably have trended downward over time as Smith and Jones refined their management of the patient population. Also over time the doctors may have been able to obtain other managed care contracts so as to achieve a larger revenue base, gain a better negotiating position in the marketplace (due to the additional membership), and achieve the inherent economics of scale associated with a larger MMHC population.

Understanding Utilization Data

In the last scenario, mistakes were made in estimating hospital utilization. This is actually a common error throughout the entire managed care field, not just in the mental health area. MMHC firms spend much energy in collecting and analyzing utilization data so as to avoid such costly mistakes. Understanding how this data is calculated and used is helpful to all concerned with managed mental health care.

The term "utilization" refers to the quantity of any particular clinical service delivered by a MMHC entity. Utilization data is sometimes expressed as a rate per 1,000 members on an annualized basis. Expressing data in this way takes fluctuating membership, or employee populations, into account and gives a meaningful picture as to how quickly treatment resources are being used.

Because hospital resources are so costly and because most MMHC groups operate with a clinical orientation of treating patients in the least restrictive setting available, utilization data relating to the use of hospital resources is key information, both from financial and clinical perspectives. As we have seen, financial miscalculations in their area can spell ruin for MMHC firms. Clinically, the over (or under) utilization of hospital resources may indicate problems in patient access, assessment, treatment, or follow-up. This data may reveal important insights into the quality of services achieved by a MMHC firm's network of community practitioners and provider hospitals.

All MMHC firms collect and scrutinize three important types of data related to inpatient care. They are *hospitalization rates*, *admission rates*, and the *average length of stay*. The most important statistic is the first, which is the rate at which members are utilizing hospital resources.

As an example, suppose a MMHC firm has 100,000 members for which it must provide or purchase all clinical services. In the month of January its members utilize 200 bed days in psychiatric or substance abuse hospitals. Its members are using hospital days, on an annual basis, at 24 days per 1,000 members. If this rate continues throughout the rest of the year members will use, and the MMHC firm will purchase on their behalf 2,400 hospital days! The formula used to arrive at this number is:

$$\frac{\text{\# hospital days used per month}}{\text{\# of capitated members}} \times 12{,}000 = \frac{\text{rate}}{1{,}000 \text{ members (annualized)}}$$

$$\text{or}$$

$$\frac{200 \text{ days used}}{100{,}000 \text{ members}} \times 12{,}000 = \frac{24}{1{,}000 \text{ members}}$$

By multiplying 24 days by 100 (the number of thousands of members) the figure of 2,400 is reached as a projection of how many hospital days will be utilized in the course of the year (assuming a stable membership).

By April the MMHC entity in this example notices a change in its hospitalization patterns. Only 100 hospital days were used by its 100,000 members in that month. Its utilization rate drops to 12 days/1,000 members, or:

$$\frac{100 \text{ days used}}{100,000 \text{ members}} \times 12,000 = \frac{12}{1,000 \text{ members}}$$

It now appears the firm will not need to purchase as many hospital days during the course of the year as it once thought.

Such seasonal variations in hospitalization needs are common and MMHC firms budget for them. They give close scrutiny to this key utilization indicator since one day in a hospital may cost the MMHC firm $500 to $1,000 or more. If the firm underestimates its hospital utilization rate and budgeting funds accordingly, a shortfall of thousands of dollars may result.

Continuing the example above and estimating each hospital day to cost $500, if the MMHC firm underestimates its hospital utilization by 25%, it will pay *one quarter million dollars* extra for its members care that year! Here is how these numbers are reached:

Projection: 20/1,000 = hospitalization rate
20 × 100 = 2,000 hospital days used in one year
20 × $500 = $1,000,000 cost of hospitalization

Actual: 25/1,000 = hospitalization rate
25 × 100 = 2,500 hospital days used in one year
2,500 × $500 = $1,250,000 cost of hospitalization

Actual Cost   = $1,250,000
Projected Cost = $1,000,000
Budget Shortfall = $250,000

MMHC firms routinely achieve hospitalization rates in the range of 20 to 50 days per 1,000 members. When these figures are contrasted with unmanaged systems where mental health and substance abuse hospitalization rates are usually in the range of 100 to 200 days per 1,000 members, it is easy to understand the rapid proliferation of MMHC! MMHC firms use their powerful data to good effect in their sales efforts since it is highly objective information and is in such sharp contrast to unmanaged care data.

The second key inpatient related statistic is the hospital admission rate, which is also expressed as a rate per 1,000 members. This statistic indicates the rate at which members are being admitted to hospitals. The same formula is used to find this rate as in the case of the hospitalization rate.

Suppose the 100,000 member firm had 12 admissions in one month. This equals to 1.44 admissions/1,000 members annually or:

$$\frac{\text{\# of admissions in one month}}{\text{\# of capitated members}} \times 12{,}000 = \text{admissions per 1,000 members, annualized}$$

or

$$\frac{12}{100{,}000} \times 12{,}000 = 1.44 \text{ per 1,000 members, annualized}$$

The third important inpatient category of data is the *Average Length of Stay* (ALOS), or how long a typical hospitalization lasts. For example, if 12 admissions in one month used 100 hospital bed days, the ALOS would be 8.33 days ($100 \div 12 = 8.33$). Firms can monitor their data separately for mental health and substance abuse clients, or as a combined statistic. MMHC organizations study which physicians and hospitals achieve the shortest ALOS for similar patients. In this way the data can help them select the most effective and efficient providers and hospitals.

MMHC firms are interested in similar utilization data about their outpatient services. They wish to understand how quickly members are presenting for care (outpatient admissions per 1,000 members), how long members are in treatment (number of sessions per treatment episode) and the rate at which members are using services (services per 1,000 members, annualized). This information can be found by using the above formulas, but substituting the appropriate outpatient data for the inpatient numbers.

For example, if the 100,000 members of our hypothetical MMHC firm used 1,250 units of outpatient services (individual, family, group, medication therapy, etc.) in one month, the rate at which services were used was 150 per 1,000 members annually. This means the firm should have the financial and clinical resources available to accommodate the delivery of 150 outpatient services for each 1,000 of its members over the course of a year. The formula used to calculate this number is:

$$\frac{\text{\# services or visits in one month}}{\text{\# of capitated members}} \times 12{,}000 = \frac{\text{rate of services used per}}{\text{1,000 members (annualized)}}$$

or

$$\frac{1{,}250}{100{,}000} \times 12{,}000 = 150 \text{ per 1,000 members, annualized}$$

MMHC operations vary, but outpatient utilization in the range of 150 services or visits per 1,000 members annually is common.

Summary

MMHC firms are usually funded through capitated arrangements. Frequently they carry the total financial risk for all contracted clinical services for their members. They carefully estimate utilization for a prospective member population which, along with the type of services called for within the proposed contract, drives the capitation rate charged to the customer. From this monthly revenue, the MMHC firm purchases or provides services to its members, pays its overhead costs, and derives an income for itself.

Poor management of the MMHC firm or factors beyond its control, such as rapidly fluctuating HMO membership, can result in financial difficulties. The outcome can be disruption in client care and hardships for the MMHC firm's providers. Adequate planning, flexibility, and substantial financial resources are needed to avoid such pitfalls.

Understanding how MMHC firms measure and analyze key utilization is important in understanding their overall operations. Key among this data is the hospitalization rate. MMHC firms usually achieve rates in the 20 to 50 days per 1,000 member range, in contrast to the 100 to 200 day range for unmanaged mental health and substance abuse care.

THE MARKET FOR MANAGED MENTAL HEALTH CARE

Managed Mental Health Care (MMHC) firms have been a fast developing business since the mid 1980s. They have come about in response to the need of HMOs and self-insured employer groups for specialty organizations to manage mental health and substance abuse benefits. These firms have rapidly become an indispensable part of the health care industry — so much so that insurance industry giants, with interstate chains of HMOs, have acquired their own specialty firms to service their health care plans and sell to employer accounts.

In 1989 CIGNA purchased Minneapolis-based MCC Companies, Inc. (Metropolitan Clinic of Counseling) to provide mental health and substance abuse management for its twenty-nine HMOs, as well as the additional plans CIGNA obtained when it purchased EQUICOR Health Plans in 1990. Founded by a clinician in the mid 1970s, MCC grew rapidly in the late 1980s providing both MMHC and employee assistance programming.

Human Affairs International (HAI) of Salt Lake City, Utah was also purchased during the same time period by AETNA to manage its HMO's mental health and substance abuse benefits. Like MCC companies, HAI was founded in the 1970s by a clinician and evolved into a leader in the 1970s and 1980s growth field of EAPs. Like CIGNA, AETNA moved in 1990 to expand its system of HMOs by completing a buy-out of PARTNER'S Health Plans.

Another industry leader is American PsychManagement (APM), based in Arlington, Virginia. As mentioned, APM successfully competed for the landmark national contract with IBM. The five year agreement, which began in July, 1990, "carves out" IBM's mental health and substance abuse benefits from their medical benefits plans across the nation. APM will provide mental health and substance abuse care to over 650,000 beneficiaries through a national provider network. Robert E. Petricelli, President of Value

Health, Inc. (APM's parent company), said that "IBM's decision
to carve out mental health treatment . . . sends a strong, positive
signal about the value of specialty managed care arrangements."

IBM's decision to turn to a MMHC firm to manage its employees' care will likely have far reaching effects. Undoubtedly IBM's
move will be emulated by other large employers. With far-flung
work forces, employers such as IBM represent a huge market for
these and other MMHC firms which operate on a national scale.

This view was recently endorsed by a Metropolitan Life survey
of insurance brokers and employee benefits consultants who are key
players in the health care field. A resounding 97% said they believed that managed care organizations would grow throughout the
decade of the 1990s.

The further development of managed care systems in the 1990s
seems consistent with the plans and attitudes expressed in a William
M. Mercer, Inc. survey of the chief executive officers of the nation's five thousand largest employers. Mercer is one of the largest
employee benefit consulting firms and conducted a survey of executive attitudes about health care costs in 1985 and again in 1990. The
1990 Mercer survey found that 92%, compared to 84% in 1985,
believed America faces a crisis in health care delivery. When questioned about approaches they employ (or plan to implement) to control health care costs for their workers, a majority endorsed such
managed care strategies as: utilization review, the encouragement
of HMOs or other alternative delivery systems, the negotiation of
reduced fees from providers, increased cost-sharing by employees,
and the restriction of reimbursement for "unnecessary" care.
Alarmingly some 60% of the Mercer survey CEOs said they have or
are considering the reduction of health care coverage as a strategy!

The message from this data is clear. America's chief executive
officers are alarmed at escalating costs for health care and are positively inclined to utilize strategies to manage these costs that are
consistent with MMHC approaches. Also, in their quest to control
costs, they are not averse to reducing benefits as means of achieving
this objective. By helping employer's achieve cost-savings,
MMHC firms may be able to preserve employer-sponsored benefits
for mental health and substance abuse treatment.

Essentially then, two markets exist for MMHC entities. One is the nation's six hundred-plus HMOs. In this area, the parent companies of the larger interstate HMO chains are acquiring or building their own specialty MMHC firms. These firms will service their own health care plans while competing for other HMO business as well. The second, larger market is self-insured (fully at risk) employers who need better management of mental health and substance abuse benefits. This market has only recently become aware of this need. It now seems likely that these employers will increasingly eliminate their MH/SA coverage with insurance carriers and HMOs, and like IBM, hire MMHC firms to help them pursue the dual goals of providing adequate mental health care for their employees, while reducing unnecessary or unduly costly care.

TRENDS

Growth

The most apparent trend is the growth of managed care systems, especially among large, self-insured employers. Widespread agreement among many authorities supports this notion. Given employers' and insurers' view that management of benefits is the best way to contain costs and prevent abuse and waste, it is likely that attitudes among practitioners in the mental health field will change. Managed care may well be seen as the only institution that can preserve benefits for consumers. Without this management, many payors may simply be unable to offer mental health and substance abuse benefit plans. In the practice environment of the 1990s, not only will most clinicians be participants in managed care systems, they will also have a large stake in its success—both in the interests of their clients and patients and their own professional futures. Those who practice treatment interventions aimed at the restoration of normal functioning, who are able to contain their operating costs, who are able to document the effectiveness of their services, who are able to demonstrate client satisfaction with their interventions, and who develop innovative marketing approaches toward managed care firms, or design and market managed care products themselves, will find the 1990s to be a rewarding practice environment.

New Systems and Applications

Managed mental health care is still in its infancy. It will continue to evolve in coming years. Clinicians, administrators, consultants, and human resource managers must continue to stay abreast of its evolution, influencing its development when possible.

Whereas much of MMHC's focus in the 1980s was on controlling skyrocketing hospitalization rates and costs, focus may shift in the 1990s to managing outpatient and office practices. As in the case of hospitals, outpatient clinicians will increasingly find it necessary to affiliate with a managed care provider network, receiving referrals through these systems. While new managed care products may evolve that offer more choice to the consumer, the choice will have a price tag which will be greater out-of-pocket expenses. This will motivate consumers to utilize such "network providers." MMHC will monitor these outpatient providers to ensure cost-conscious and effective care.

Treatment Orientation

Clinicians will increasingly be influenced to utilize interventions aimed at the restoration of normal functioning, not personality change or the restructuring of long-standing personality styles. Clinicians will need increased familiarity with short-term, brief therapy techniques and interventions, which are philosophically compatible with managed care values and benefit constraints. Opportunities will proliferate for clinicians who are able to develop innovative workplace counseling services aimed at maintaining healthy work forces. Other opportunities will exist for new programs and services aimed at treating acute patients outside of hospital walls and preventing rehospitalization. This includes after-hours crisis intervention services and home-based psychiatric treatment programs.

Academia will be challenged to respond to the development of managed care systems by modifying curriculums to include more information about these systems and their impact on clinical practice. Joseph Steiner, PhD, a social work educator at Syracuse University says graduate students are eager to learn about managed care delivery systems and its implication for their careers. "Many want to understand how it will affect the private practice environment and their futures as clinicians," says Steiner, who teaches seminars on managed care themes. He also believes that academicians should become more involved in outcome research which will better guide managed care decision-makers and practitioners alike in developing cost-effective treatment interventions (Personal communication, 1990).

Educators and researchers will also likely investigate many issues related to solution-focused treatments and other techniques that are aimed at rapid change in clients. Understanding the types of problems most amenable to remediation in one or two visits has importance to MMHC and EAP practitioners alike. Research concerning these and other managed care-related themes will be an important contribution by academia in the coming years.

The Increased Role of Automated Systems

The role that electronic automated systems play in practice will increase. An example of this is Prudential Insurance Company's plan to install, by the end of 1991, terminals in the offices of primary care physicians in its forty-three managed care networks across the United States. These terminals, similar to the familiar grocery store check-out devices, will be used to instantly verify benefits and produce claims information.

With this system, developed by Health Information Technologies of Princeton, New Jersey, the benefit card is passed through the terminal, or if the member has no card, the identification number is entered. In a few seconds the enrollee's eligibility is verified, benefits are displayed, as well as the status of deductibles, copayments and needed precertification or authorization information. Other insurance and managed care firms are planning to implement this or similar systems in the near future to help providers better access information.

Quoted in a recent edition of Health Week, Prudential spokesman Tom Joyce said, "We're making a mélange of managed care products easier for doctors to administer." Physicians can also use the system to simplify claims filing. Such advances will first come to the physician offices of managed care networks and then to the offices of nonphysician clinicians. Group or clinic style practices will be the first to benefit from this technology of convenience, as cost may initially make such systems prohibitative for small, solo practices.

Automated scheduling systems will also become more common. These systems will allow centralized EAP or UR firms to instantly schedule appointments for clients in any one of a large number of clinic or network provider offices. Automation will simplify the authorization and claims filing processes, reducing paper flow.

Nationalized Health Care and Public Policy

Some have questioned whether or not a nationalized health care system, if ever implemented, would supplant managed care technologies and offer an alternative solution to America's health care crisis. Should such a system be developed, it would likely feature more, not fewer managed care procedures. Its managers would continue to be confronted with identical quality of care and access issues, while managing taxpayers' resources to finance the massive endeavor.

Meanwhile, industry leaders say that less, not more government control is needed in the future. According to CIGNA Chairman and Chief Executive Officer Bill Taylor the delivery of quality, affordable health care can be achieved through enhancing the private-public partnership that exists today. "It can be done without further government intervention, centralization, or additional financing. What is needed first is to make both the private and public sides of the health care equation work more cost-effectively through available managed care techniques," Taylor said in a recent address to the National Association of Manufacturers. He pointed to integrated health care plans as means of achieving affordable, quality health care. He cited the experience of corporate giant Allied-Signal, who reduced the cost of financing health services $750 per employee during an eighteen month period while utilizing such a plan. Allied-Signal expects to save more than $200 million over three years. Taylor encouraged government to apply managed care systems to Medicare and Medicaid (CIGNA, 1990).

Public policy may be reshaped in the future to accommodate

more aspects of managed care technology within existing mental health and substance abuse service delivery systems. Community mental health centers, too frequently characterized by long waiting lists for services, may benefit from the treatment approaches favored by MMHC. The introduction of short-term interventions aimed at restoration of normal functioning, not characterological change may aid in eliminating these waiting lists for outpatient treatment for many clients. At the same time, better management of scarce public hospital resources, through the use of managed care-originated procedures, may well serve the chronically mentally ill populations. Public sector clinicians, administrators, planners, and policy makers will examine managed care systems closely in coming years in an effort to glean their best features and approaches, and to determine how to modify and apply them to public settings.

REFERENCES

Berk, M. L., Monheit, A. C., & Hagan, M. M. (1988, Fall). How the U.S. spent its health care dollar, 1929-1980. *Health Affairs*, pp. 46-60.

Bistline, J. L. (November 1990). Personal communication.

Bistline, J. L., Sheridan, S. M., & Winegar, N. (1991). Five critical skills for mental health counselors in managed health care. *Journal of Mental Health Counseling, 13* (1), 147-152.

CIGNA. (1990, December). Quality, affordable health care possible for all Americans. *Cigna News*, p. 1.

Cummings, N. A. (1986). The dismantling of our health care systems: Strategies for the survival of psychological practice. *American Psychologist, 41*, 426-431.

Julius, D. (1990, October). Personal communication.

LaPensee, K. T. (1991). Mental health benefits: What are the real needs and how can we control costs? In *Driving down health care costs: Strategies and solutions* (pp. 11-1//nd11-13). New York: Panel Publishers, Inc.

Levin, B. L., & Glasser, J. H. (1989). Mental health service coverage within prepaid health plans. *Administration in Mental Health, 7*, 271-281.

Mullen, P. (1990, December 7). Prudential preps electronic claims verification. *Health Week*, p. 9.

Pigott, H. E. (1990). Psychiatric home health care: One prescription for soaring mental health costs. In *Driving down health care costs: Strategies and solutions* (pp. 9-1//nd9-10). New York: Panel Publishers, Inc.

Shadle, M., & Christianson, J. B. (1989). The impact of HMO development on mental health and chemical dependency services. *Hospital and Community Psychiatry, 40*, 1145-1151.

Shadle, M., & Christianson, J. B. (1988). The organization of mental health care delivery in HMO's. *Administration in Mental Health*, *15*, 201-225.

Staff. (1990, August-September). Insurance brokers see managed care growing. *AMCRA Newsletter*, p. 6.

Staff. (1990, August-September). Largest managed mental health care contract awarded. *AMCRA Newsletter*, p. 6.

Wagman, J. B. & Schif, J. (1990). Managed mental health care for employees: Roles for social workers. In *Occupational Social Work Today* (pp. 53-66). New York: The Haworth Press.

William M. Mercer, Inc. (1991). Employer attitudes toward the cost of health care—1990. In *Driving down health care costs: Strategies and solutions* (pp. 15-1//nd15-18). New York: Panel Publishers, Inc.

Winegar, N., Bistline, J. L., & Sheridan, S. M. (in press). Quality and cost-effectiveness: Establishing a group therapy program in a managed care setting. *Families in Society*.

Chapter Six

Managing
the Utilization Management Process

Utilization management (UM) in MMHC systems refers to any of several techniques and procedures used to monitor and evaluate the necessity or appropriateness of care for insurance coverage or provider reimbursement purposes. UM ensures that services delivered are appropriate and necessary and are authorized in advance for reimbursement. UM decisions are based on information concerning clients that includes symptoms, diagnostic impressions, tentative treatment plans, response to treatment and treatment outcomes.

UM is a term, like several others in the managed care arena, that means different things to different people. It is widely perceived as one of the most controversial areas in managed mental health care. At best, it helps to ensure that care given to consumers is needed and appropriate and that the provider of this care will indeed be reimbursed for services rendered. At worst, UM is perceived as an undue intrusion into the client-therapist relationship, one that is driven by cost reduction at the expense of quality of care. Since UM procedures have demonstrated an ability to reduce hospitalization utilization, its most vocal critics are often hospitals and hospital-affiliated providers who are accustomed to inpatient-based treatment for many patients.

TYPES OF UM PROCEDURES

UM functions may be carried out in one of several ways. Telephonic UM may be conducted by local clinicians or through large centralized operations. Advantages to local UM include a better knowledge by the UM staff of local resources and providers, as well as a better opportunity to develop satisfactory working relationships with provider colleagues. Centralized UM affords cost savings due to the reduced expense of operations since one center eliminates the need for numerous locations. Mental health related utilization management may be provided by MMHC firms or by EAPs.

UM may also be provided through on-site interviews, similar to how some HMOs conduct medical/surgical UM. In this example, the UM clinician might visit a hospital, interview the patient or provider(s), and read the clinical record in order to obtain first-hand information.

In MMHC systems, UM functions may be the responsibility of one staff member, or they may be diffused throughout several clinicians. In medical/surgical settings, either in HMOs or in utilization management firms, UM is typically provided by nurses and physicians. However in MMHC systems, other clinicians such as psychologists, clinical social workers, professional counselors and other qualified mental health professionals may conduct UM activities. Psychiatrists are utilized directly in oversight and supervisory capacities. UM may be applied to both outpatient and inpatient cases, and UM activities, especially precertification for admission, are provided twenty-four hours per day by MMHC entities.

The key task in UM procedures involves the collection of adequate clinical information needed to determine if potential or proposed services for any particular case are necessary and are eligible for reimbursement under the individual's health care or benefit plan. Alternatives may be suggested by the UM clinician if the original proposed treatment was determined to be unnecessary or not a covered service.

The core functions of UM are described below.

Eligibility Determination

Eligibility determination is a UM function that ensures that any member is indeed a valid member and is eligible for covered services. This is usually done electronically.

Benefit Interpretation

Benefit interpretation is an important aspect of UM in which the MMHC clinician determines whether the presenting condition is one that is eligible for covered services.

Precertification for Admission

Precertification for admission (or "pre-cert") refers to UM personnel making the above determination *before* an individual is admitted to an inpatient facility or an outpatient episode of treatment. Care is then authorized for reimbursement in advance or alternative (usually less costly) care is recommended. (See Figure 6-1.) An example of how this precertification process works is described below.

Mr. Black is a fifty-year-old, married engineer who receives health insurance coverage through his employer's plan. His drinking problem has gradually accelerated over the years. He has never sought treatment, and never attended Alcoholics Anonymous. On a Sunday morning, after a particularly painful episode of drinking, his wife, who is familiar with Recovery Hospital's substance abuse treatment program, convinces her husband to go there and seek services. The admission nurse at the hospital accesses the UM clinician associated with Mr. Black's health care plan by dialing the twenty-four-hour number on the benefit card Mr. Black presented. The UM clinician obtained clinical data from the admissions nurse and Mr. and Mrs. Black. The UM clinician (after consulting with her physician back-up) determines that the proposed twenty-eight-day hospitalization for alcoholism is not clinically necessary, and that an alternative form of treatment will be appropriate and will be covered by the health care plan. The clinician recommends instead an intensive outpatient treatment program, after a screening by Mr. Black's physician. The new plan is discussed with the patient and his wife. He begins the treatment program authorized the next night, having also returned to work.

Although this vignette is a simplified one it illustrates several important features of precertification:

Accessibility, twenty-four-hour, 365-day per year accessibility is required of UM functions. Psychiatric and substance abuse crises

FIGURE 6-1. Precertification for Admissions

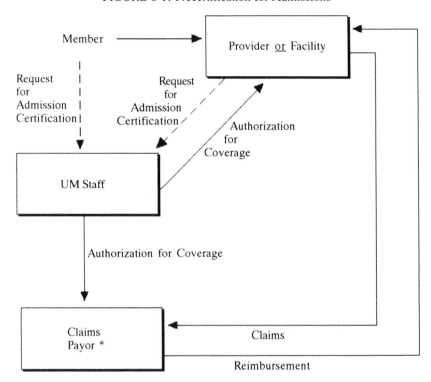

*This entity may be the MMHC firm, the HMO, insurance carrier, or another party functioning as a Third Party Administrator (TPA)

occur at all hours, so MMHC systems must have easily accessible UM capacity at all times.

Consultation and medical backup, often through a supervising psychiatrist, are important resources to the UM clinician. In the example above, the clinician collected available data about Mr. Black's medical condition both from the hospital's admission worker and the patient. The determination was made that Mr. Black was in no immediate danger from acute alcohol withdrawal symptoms. While treatment at the hospital may have offered the maximum level and intensity of care, the patient was able to participate in an alternative, less costly level of care.

Crisis nature of precertification situations. Such precertification processes may be conducted in the midst of an emotion-laden series of events. In this instance, both the patient and his spouse as well as the admission worker may have attempted to persuade the UM clinician to authorize care in the hospital setting. At that moment admission to the facility was viewed as a crucial need. This well intended pressure did not prevent the worker from collecting necessary clinical information and making the decision about precertification. In other words the UM clinician had to deny the request for coverage in such a way as to maintain a therapeutic contract with the member and maintain a working relationship with the hospital personnel. Much clinical expertise was needed to frame the hospital presentation by the Blacks as an important milestone and refocus their attention toward outpatient treatment avenues.

Cost savings. In a system without precertification (where essentially the admission worker in this example would have obtained coverage simply by facilitating the admission) the cost of Mr. Black's twenty-eight days of treatment might have been $14,000 or more. Most of the cost would have been borne by the health care plan. Instead, the patient was directed to a treatment program costing only $2,000 over the course of one year. Additionally, the patient continued working. The cost savings amounted to $12,000 directly, and much more in indirect savings to the plan and the member.

Concurrent Review

As implied, this review occurs concurrently with the treatment service provided to MMHC members. It assesses the need for continued treatment in a hospital setting or continuation with a course of outpatient treatment. (See Figure 6-2.)

In instances of hospital concurrent review, the UM clinician often will authorize one day or a few days coverage initially. After the inpatient has been assessed, a prospective discharge date is established between the UM clinician and attending physician. Further hospital coverage may be authorized pending the determination of a tentative D/C date. Periodic telephonic updates are used to monitor the patient's progress throughout the hospital stay and obtain and

FIGURE 6-2. Concurrent Review

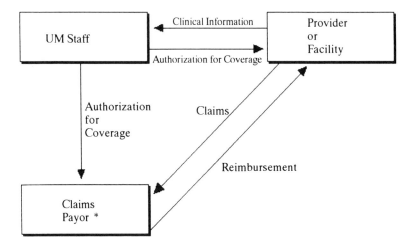

*This entity may be the MMHC firm, the HMO, insurance carrier, or another party functioning as a Third Party Administrator (TPA)

evaluate any new clinical information that might lengthen or shorten the duration of the necessary hospital care.

UM staff play an active role in discharge planning and clinical case management for inpatients. Discharge planning on the part of the MMHC firm is likely to begin at the time of hospital admission. The UM clinician may present the case in a clinical staffing or team meeting. Treatment modalities and community resources are reviewed. Often the family is interviewed. The UM clinician becomes the liaison with hospital staff in efforts to coordinate this planning and a smooth transition to outpatient treatment.

In systems that utilize a DRG reimbursement system for hospital stabilization, treatment, or detoxification, the concurrent role is de-emphasized. Activity by the UM staff is more focused in the area of discharge planning, since DRGs tend to affix in advance a discharge date for many patients.

Outpatient concurrent review processes begin with an authorization for coverage for "X" number of visits. The initial precertification and authorization may occur after the MMHC firm has conducted an initial assessment, after the treatment provider has conducted the assessment and communicated it to the UM clinician, or in some cases, after another clinician who will not provide treatment services has evaluated the member. Authorizations are typically mailed to the member as well as the provider. Much outpatient concurrent review is done through the use of various written updates and summaries. These communicate to the UM staff how the authorized treatment is progressing and how the patient responded to the services. Appendix C shows samples of such concurrent review authorizations, forms, and letters. The following case study demonstrates the application of several UM techniques.

Ms. Ferguson is twenty-six years old, and employed as an accountant. She presented at the office of her primary care physician, who contacted the UM staff at the MMHC. She was assessed by the UM staff as exhibiting severe depressive symptomatology. An admission was precertified at a nonnetwork psychiatric hospital and three days were authorized initially. Initial treatment goals included further assessment and symptom stabilization.

On the third day telephone concurrent review was conducted between the UM staff and the treating psychiatrist. The patient had been diagnosed with major depression, single episode. The psychiatrist indicated that the patient, who had been started on a course of antidepressant medication on the day of admission, had demonstrated little response to the medication or the hospital milieu. She judged that the patient could not be treated safely as an outpatient until further stabilization occurred. The psychiatrist stated that further care could provide close observation of her medication response and provide a safe environment. She also requested coverage for a session with the patient and her spouse to address marital dysfunction, which seemed to be exacerbating the depression. The psychiatrist indicated she planned to discuss with the patient and her husband outpatient treatment services which would follow inpatient care. Three additional days were authorized with a tentative discharge date being established for the seventh day.

The UM clinician contacted the psychiatrist on the day before the tentative discharge. The psychiatrist reported the patient had responded favorably, and the outpatient plan for services was confirmed. The attending psychiatrist conveyed that Ms. Ferguson's condition had stabilized enough for her to make the transition to outpatient care. Her depressive symptoms had diminished and the lethality risk had declined. The psychiatrist recommended that medication therapy be continued and counseling services initiated with the couple. Ms. Ferguson was seen the day of discharge by the MMHC affiliated providers in the outpatient setting.

The case of Ms. Ferguson illustrates several important qualities about inpatient concurrent review. Care is authorized for treatment interventions which are implemented at the onset of the hospital stay. Authorization for coverage of subsequent days is based on specific clinical data regarding the patient's response and progress, and care is expected to be focused towards specific objectives. Another quality illustrated is that discharge planning begins early in the hospital stay. Finally, the working relationship with the attending physician is key. The psychiatrist shared the objectives of the UM staff of stabilizing the patient's condition as quickly as possible and preparing Ms. Ferguson for outpatient treatment as soon as appropriate.

TYPICAL UM QUESTIONS

UM decisions are based on clinical data obtained through the means previously discussed. Below are generalized UM questions which may be used to gather the necessary clinical information. In practice, more specific details are usually elicited.

- What is the member's DSM-III-R diagnosis(es)?
- How, or by what means, was this diagnosis reached?
- What is the member's current mental status and lethality?
- What, if any, treatment history is known? (i.e., number of hospitalizations, length of prior hospital stays, number of outpatient visits)
- What alternative types of treatment have been considered for this member?
- What are the clinical goals for this treatment episode?
- How will more treatment (more hospital days or visits) contribute to achieving these goals?
- How will treatment outcomes, i.e., the achievement of particular goals, be measured?

MEDICAL NECESSITY

The determination of what care or treatment is medically necessary is the central consideration in precertification and concurrent review decisions. Clinical information gathered by UM staff is aimed at this question. The responsibility for making this decision as it pertains to benefit coverage is delegated to the MMHC from the firm's customer, an HMO or employer. This issue has been, and will continue to be, the focus of litigation and court rulings. (See Chapter Seven for further discussion of the legal underpinning of UM decisions related to the necessity.)

UM staff are guided by what medically necessary care means in mental health or substance abuse settings through standards or treatment criteria utilized to authorize care for respective diagnoses. These standards do not represent "cookbooks," they instead are guides requiring clinical interpretation and application on a care-by-care basis (*Clinical Psychiatry News*, 1990).

In the vignette of Mr. Black, the UM criteria in operation helped the clinician arrive at an authorization decision by determining that:

a. the member was not a medical risk for alcohol withdrawal complications necessitating twenty-four hour nursing care;
b. the member was in need of treatment and was motivated for treatment;
c. the member had never attempted outpatient substance abuse treatment.

Therefore, outpatient substance abuse treatment was recommended to him and was authorized for coverage by his health care plan.

MCC Companies, Inc., which has both centralized and local market UM capabilities, has developed a *Preferred Practice Guide* (1989), which outlines practice standards for the treatment of various disorders. MCC continues to refine and revise it in an effort to assist its UM operations concerning these determinations. Application of such documents helps to ensure MMHC customers consistency and uniformity where multiple sites are involved. Although professional groups such as the American Psychiatric Association are now developing standards of treatment documents, the historic lack of such standards and a consensus about them among various professionals has led to the development of MMHC. In effect the payors, through MMHC firms, have driven the development treatment standards themselves.

DENIALS, APPEALS, AND OTHER UM ASPECTS

All MMHC firms have appeal processes to review UM decisions that have resulted in a denial of authorization for coverage. These procedures may require a written appeal, others involved an "expedited appeal process" by which a decision about the appeal may take place while the disputed care is still underway. Quality utilization management firms have clear procedures for these expedited or emergent appeals. UM processes usually involve a physician's approval in cases where a requested authorization (especially hospitalization) is denied.

Often, UM staff will offer to retrospectively review a disputed request. This offer implies that coverage for services may be extended retroactively, pending the review. This review process includes the examination of complete treatment records as well as other supplemental materials. UM staff typically advise providers and members in writing of denials for coverage.

MMHC clinicians also apply UM procedures to psychological assessment and evaluations. Not all psychological testing may be covered by a MMHC benefit plan, and testing is preauthorized. UM staff frequently authorize testing for the following reasons:

a. To clarify a diagnostic impression. Providers who are unsure of a diagnosis may be authorized to conduct particular assessments to establish or rule out a diagnosis.
b. To focus treatment. Providers who request specific tests that will help establish appropriate treatment goals may have testing authorized by UM staff.

Generally, MMHC UM standards do not include routine authorizations for complete psychological evaluations for every client. Again, UM staff view testing as a resource to be authorized for coverage on an as-needed basis, usually centering around the criteria above.

The confidentiality of client information obtained through UM processes is assumed by the provider-MMHC agreement. (See the sample agreement in Appendix A). However, it is wise to obtain a signed authorization for disclosures to the MMHC or UM firm and to fully explain to a client that information about his or her treatment is being reported for reimbursement of services rendered.

Provider-UM staff relationships have great potential for difficulty, but it is not necessary that this be the case. Here are some tips on how to create this problematic relationship and how to diffuse it.

Twelve Strategies for Creating Problematic Relationship with UM Staff . . . And Alternatives!

Strategy No. 1:   Never use the DSM III-R diagnostic system and nomenclature.

Alternative: Become familiar with the DSM III-R diagnostic system and nomenclature. Be prepared to document your diagnosis and communicate it to the UM staff.

Strategy No. 2:   Establish vague, or no, treatment goals with the client (and do so slowly).

Alternative: Join with the client in establishing achievable, mutually agreed upon goals quickly. Use a written treatment plan. Clarify goals early in the assessment and treatment process.

Strategy No. 3:   Establish vague, or no, outcome measures for any treatment goals (and do so slowly).

Alternative: Develop with the client what outcome measures of the treatment goals will be utilized. Be concise, concrete, and as behaviorally oriented as possible. Be able to explain to UM personnel exactly how you will know when the client has achieved agreed upon goals for the treatment episode.

Strategy No. 4:   Keep vague, or no, clinical notes. Reconstruct important issues about therapy sessions from memory for the UM staff.

Alternative: Keep accurate written notes about all clinical contacts with the client. The S.O.A.P. format, or a variation, is an excellent means of accomplishing this documentation. (See Appendix D.) The ability to access these notes and provide documentation of progress or setbacks is vital to successful working relationships with UM personnel.

Strategy No. 5:   Play "telephone-tag" with the UM staff conducting concurrent review. After a few tries, give up!

Alternative: Schedule a time of day and/or day of the week to discuss cases with the UM staff doing concurrent review. This simplifies your task and theirs.

Strategy No. 6:   Remain as ignorant as possible of the MMHC firm's standards for treatment.

Alternative: Ask the UM staff of the MMHC firm to share information about their standards of care. Learn what the preferred types and durations of treatment are for particular diagnostic groups, realizing the need for case-by-case variations.

Strategy No. 7:   Assume "precertification" or "preauthorization" does not really mean "*pre*." Call the MMHC firm's UM staff long after the client has been admitted for services.

Alternative: Precertification and preauthorization mean, for reimbursement purposes, that services must be authorized *in advance*. Not obtaining such advance authorization for benefit coverage can mean the financial responsibility for services may fall upon the provider or the client.

Strategy No. 8:   Interpret the client's benefits yourself. Interpret them as liberally as you wish, including the conditions you feel *should* be included for coverage in the benefit plan. Express any resentments about benefit limits, exclusions, or UM processes through the client.

Alternative: Do not interpret benefits to the client. This responsibility has been delegated to the MMHC firm by the purchaser of benefits, the HMO, or the employer. Refer benefit questions to the UM staff. Do not express resentments or concerns through the client. This is counter-therapeutic. Express concerns about benefit limits or how they are interpreted directly to the MMHC firm, employer, or through avenues such as professional associations.

Strategy No. 9:   Do not bother about learning the MMHC firm's appeal process for reversing UM decisions.

Alternative: Learn about this appeal process, and how and when to use it. Upon appeal, UM decisions are sometimes reversed. Learn about the UM firm's expedited appeal procedure.

Strategy No. 10:   Do not bother with UM related paperwork. If you do, do so incompletely and slowly.

Alternative: The paperwork related to UM is a necessary fact of practice. It is important for accountability purposes and ignoring it will be problematic. Complete it as expeditiously as possible. Suggest ways to streamline the necessary paperwork or develop alternative ways of processing the paper flow.

Strategy No. 11:   Expect only stable, nonacute referrals from UM staff; expect UM staff to authorize coverage for maximal treatment interventions and durations.

Alternative: Anticipate receiving acute clients with the expectation on the part of the UM staff that the provider will initiate treatment quickly. Expect authorization for care that is not necessarily the maximal intervention, but one that the UM staff has deemed appropriate to the degree of need and that will return the client to normal levels of functioning as soon as possible. Expect the UM staff to be driven by values of efficiency, effectiveness, and cost-consciousness.

Strategy No. 12:   Assume that UM staff are excessively rigid and unlikely to be open to innovation. Approach them by evidencing these qualities yourself.

Alternative: UM staff can be very flexible and innovative. Both they and the MMHC firm are interested in exploring innovative programs, services, and arrangements for providing clinically effective and cost-effective assessment and treatment services. Approach UM staff with the intent of forming a mutually satisfactory partnership aimed at providing quality services for both customers: the client and the MMHC firm.

REFERENCES

Bartlett, J. (Ed.). (1990). *Preferred practice guide*. Minneapolis, MN: MCC Managed Behavioral Care, Inc.

Gray, B. H., & Field, M. J. (Eds.). (1990). *Controlling costs and changing patient care: The role of utilization management*. Washington, DC: National Academy Press.

(1990, November). Need to develop flexible practice guidelines emphasized. *Clinical Psychiatry News*, p. 9.

Chapter Seven

Legal Issues
and Utilization Management

MAJOR CASES

Utilization management (UM) systems can substantially impact the delivery of care. Therefore, UM decisions have the potential for harm to consumers and are subject to legal liabilities. The issues surrounding the exact nature and extent of such liabilities are complex, and are unfolding both through case law and the implementation of new legislation and regulation. It is beyond the scope of this discussion to detail and explore all the intricacies of this topic. Instead, this chapter will focus on major cases in recent years that have been construed as establishing the legal underpinnings of the UM process.*

The first case was that of *Sarchett*, which upheld the right of an insurer to participate in the decision making and determination of what care is "medically necessary" and therefore reimbursable. The *Wickline* case dealt with the liability potential of the UM organization resulting from the possibility of harm to the patient as an outcome of a UM decision. Both are medical/surgical cases, but their implications transcend to managed mental health UM as well. The *Wilson* case has not been disposed of by the courts at this writing, but may ultimately have substantial implications for the utilization management field.

---

*For an excellent and fuller discussion see Helvestine, William A. (1989). "Legal Implications of Utilization Review," In Bradford H. Gray and Marilyn J. Field (Eds), *Controlling Costs and Changing Patient Care: The Role of Utilization Management*. Washington, DC: Institute of Medicine National Academy Press, pp. 169-204. Helvestine is the major source for this chapter.

Sarchett v. Blue Shield of California, 1987 (43 Cal. 3d. 1, 233 Cal. Rptr. 76, 729 p. 2d 267)

This case involved a retrospective review by an indemnity insurance company's UM staff. The plaintiff, John Sarchett, had been hospitalized for three days by his primary care physician. Later, Blue Shield UM staff reviewed the hospitalization records. They determined that (1) the hospitalization of Mr. Sarchett had been for diagnostic purposes only, and (2) the hospitalization had not been medically necessary. Their position was that it was not necessary to utilize this level of care — hospitalization — to achieve the diagnostic goals. Coverage for the charges associated with the hospitalization was denied. Blue Shield pointed out that the denial was based on two policy exclusions: (1) hospitalization for diagnostic purposes only, and (2) care that is not medically necessary. Sarchett claimed that he relied upon his physician, and the physician's judgement was that the hospital care was necessary.

The California Supreme Court held that Blue Shield could indeed perform a retrospective review, examining the medical necessity of the hospitalization. The court held that this is an implied right of an insurer. Furthermore, it rejected the premise that only the treating physician could determine medical necessity and that Blue Shield should be bound by the physician's judgement. The court endorsed the practice of preadmission certification as a means of avoiding such disputes.

The importance of *Sarchett*, then, is twofold. It helped establish the prerogative of insurance carriers, for coverage purposes, to participate in defining what care is medically necessary. Moreover, it denied that *only* the treating clinician can make this determination and bind an insurance carrier to this decision for coverage purposes.

Wickline v. California (192 Cal. App. 3d 1630, 239 Cal. Rptr. 810, 1986)

Wickline has proven to be a seminal case in the area of UM liability. It relates to the key issue of what is the extent of the UM firm's liability for poor clinical outcomes that may stem from a UM decision. The case pertains to the concurrent review process concerning the care given to a patient in 1977. The concurrent review organization was the state's Medicaid program, Medi-Cal.

The plaintiff, Mrs. Wickline, was being treated for leg and back ailments. Her physicians recommended hospitalization and surgery. Consistent with Medi-Cal's procedures, the admission was precertified. An approved length-of-stay of ten days was authorized; any stay beyond the ten days would require further authorization by Medi-Cal. The patient had complications after the first surgery, however, and two more surgeries were performed. The treating physician requested that eight more hospital days be authorized for coverage by Medi-Cal (for a total LOS of eighteen days). A Medi-Cal nurse, consulting with a Medi-Cal physician, reviewed the case again and responded to the treating physician's request with an authorization for four more days' coverage for the hospital care (for a total LOS of fourteen, not the requested eighteen days). The nurse reviewer did not document the specific reasons for the partial denial of coverage.

The physician discharged Mrs. Wickline after the authorized stay of fourteen days. (All of the physicians involved in the case were aware of the Medi-Cal appeal process, but none appealed the concurrent review decision). At the time of discharge the patient was stable and was not in danger according to subsequent court testimony. Her physician reported that the last days in the hospital were used for observation of Mrs. Wickline's condition and progress. He stated that he would have continued her hospital treatment, regardless of the Medi-Cal coverage decision, if he had felt she needed more hospital care. One week after the discharge Mrs. Wickline was seen in her physician's office for follow-up. Nothing remarkable was found. Then, nine days after discharge, Mrs. Wickline grew worse and was readmitted to a hospital. Eventually her right leg had to be amputated at the hip. Mrs. Wickline later sued Medi-Cal for negligence, alleging that Medi-Cal's decision to not authorize the additional eight hospital days requested by her physician resulted in her injury (the injury being the subsequent amputation of her right leg).

A jury trial was held in the *Wickline* case. The jury awarded the patient $500,000 in damages for her injury, but the California Court of Appeals reversed the jury verdict.

The *Wickline* case and decision involved several key issues. First, the UM firm (Medi-Cal itself in this case) was sued for negligence, the most likely cause for legal actions brought against UM firms. In order to prove negligence, the plaintiff must demonstrate that the defendant owed the plaintiff a duty of reasonable care, that the duty was not fulfilled, and that, as a result, an injury occurred. Courts have agreed that UM firms have a duty of care to patients (since nonauthorization of care may mean that the patient will not seek care), and that there must be reasonable standards of care as well as reasonable processes to apply the standards. Plaintiffs have the greatest difficulty in proving negligence when attempting to demonstrate that UM decisions are causative, i.e., result in injury that would not have otherwise occurred.

The appellate court's ruling related to these aspects of proving negligence on the part of a UM firm. First, the Court of Appeals ruled the UM organization played a role in the discharge decision, but that *ultimate responsibility for Mrs. Wickline's discharge lay with her physicians.* In other words, Medi-Cal was not proximately responsible for the decision to discharge her after fourteen days.

Secondly, the court did not find that the decision to discharge was causative of the later amputation. Mrs. Wickline's own physicians said, in effect, that she was stable when she left the hospital. Moreover, she was doing well seven days after the hospital discharge, three days beyond the hospital time originally requested for authorization.

Finally, the court held that UM groups are participants in important treatment decisions and therefore can be liable for defects of design in their systems, or for poor implementation of such systems. The decision served to put such firms on notice that their processes must be adequately designed and administered in order to reduce their liability in cases with unfortunate outcomes.

The *Wickline* decision points out to clinicians some interesting features of our judicial system. First is the difficulty of proving that any UM decision results in an injury. The plaintiff in this case was not able to show that her deterioration and subsequent amputation could have been prevented if she had been authorized for the extra four hospital days. In the realm of psychiatric and behavioral medicine, a demonstration of causation might be even more difficult to prove.

Second, the *Wickline* case clearly demonstrates the sympathetic nature of the jury system. A jury of her peers assessed that Mrs. Wickline, who presented before them as an infirmed amputee, had been wronged by the bureaucratic blunders of an uncaring, quasi-governmental insurance carrier. It easily awarded her $500,000 (only to have the decision reversed later by the appellate court). A lesson insurance companies have learned from this is to settle out of court with plaintiffs who are particularly "attractive" to sympathetic jurors, thus avoiding costly legal proceedings in jury trials and appeals courts.

Wilson v. Blue Cross of Southern California et al. (No. B04597, Cal. Ct App filed July 27, 1990)

The same division of the state court of appeals that handed down the landmark *Wickline* decision recently made another important ruling concerning a case that is unfolding. Its implications may be far reaching. In this case a patient was admitted to an inpatient facility for the treatment of depression. The physician estimated the needed length of stay as three to four weeks of hospital-based care. Blue Cross' utilization review firm informed the hospital that it would not cover the extended stay, and the patient was discharged. A few weeks later he committed suicide. His heirs then sued the insurer, the UM firm, and its physician consultant for wrongful death.

The trial court decided to grant the defendant's (Blue Cross et al.) motion for a summary judgement. The appeal court reversed this decision and remanded the case for a trial on its merits. The court held that the facts presented by the plaintiffs constituted sufficient evidence for a triable issue concerning a causal link between the denial of insurance coverage and the death of the patient a few weeks later. The court also said that the UM program's emphasis on cost containment inappropriately affected medical judgement, with a result of a premature discharge. This was in contrast to the *Wickline* case, in which the court held that the provider was responsible for the decision to discharge the patient. The ultimate outcome of *Wilson* may greatly influence UM processes.

IMPLICATIONS FOR EMPLOYERS

UM firms, their employees and consultants, and/or their insurance carrier or self-insured employer who hires them, may be brought to court concerning a range of other charges. Plaintiff's attorneys usually pursue the "deepest pocket," that is, the insurance company, the state (as in the *Wickline* case), or an employer, instead of a UM or managed care firm. Charges may involve infliction of emotional distress through a UM decision, breach of contract, product liability, or other concerns.

UM firms may also be sued by treatment providers. In *Slaughter v. Friedman* (32 Cal. 3d. 148, 185 Cal Rptr. 244, 649 p. 2d a66, 1982), the plaintiff, an oral surgeon, successfully claimed a dental insurance company's medical director defamed his professional reputation when denying claims for his services. The director had said that he was overcharging his patients. Statements such as these, when made by a UM firm to a patient, may indicate malice toward a particular provider. UM firms should be careful, for this reason, to not use unnecessarily inflammatory language to patients about providers.

Employers who attempt to contain costs for their employee benefit programs by designing their own benefit plan or by contracting with MMHC or UM firms may take several steps to limit their exposure to liability claims. Here are some strategies and examples of how they may be applied.

Although unlikely, it is possible that an employer who purchases services for employees through an HMO or PPO can have potential liability for the malpractice of the HMO or PPO sanctioned provider. (In this instance the employer's liability would be premised on negligent selection of the HMO or PPO, a difficult point to establish.) Employers can avoid this situation by selecting accredited HMOs or PPOs who have adequate credentialing policies and procedures.

Despite the protections afforded by the Employee Retirement and Income Security Act (ERISA), employers who self-insure still have the responsibility to act in the employee's best interests concerning the administration of benefits, a high standard of operation requiring close scrutiny of MMHC or UM vendors acting on the employer's behalf. Here are some steps these employers may consider to assume quality service delivery.

- Use a written selection process as a guide to selecting a MMHC/UM vendor. Follow the process.
- Use a corporate panel of appropriate staff to review and monitor the services of MMHC/UM firms. These panels may include the medical director, attorney, benefits manager, human resources manager, and Employee Assistance Program director or consultant.
- Inspect the MMHC/UM firm's credentialing process for its providers. Does the firm have adequate policies and procedures to screen out unethical or poor quality practitioners? Does it ensure that its providers have adequate malpractice insurance and that it is always current? Are its providers licensed or certified for delivering the services they intend to perform?
- Ensure that the MMHC/UM firm employs licensed and/or certified staff who practice within the scope of their licensure. Are the MMHC/UM firm's programs licensed where applicable?
- Ensure that the MMHC/UM firm bases its operations upon written clinical standards and level of care guidelines? Are these standards consistently employed? Ensure that there are adequate safeguards to prevent abuse of the standards for the financial gain of the firm.
- Educate employees about benefit plans and about their interface with the company's Employee Assistance Programs. Ensure that employees understand that benefits may be limited to medically necessary care, if this is the case.

STATE REGULATIONS AND ERISA

At the time of this writing, several states have just enacted or are proposing legislation to regulate UM processes and entities. This will likely be a trend for several years to come. State legislation in this arena pertains to obtaining a certificate to function as a UM firm application processes, confidentiality of patient records, minimum personnel qualifications, and processes for the appeal of decisions made by UM firms. It is important that clinicians and providers input into this developing legislation. Professional associations should monitor any relevant legislative initiatives.

In a 1987 case (reaffirmed in 1990) the U.S. Supreme Court ruled that when insurance is provided through a self-insured or ERISA qualified plan (see Chapter One for a fuller description of ERISA) state law is preempted by ERISA. Most private employers' plans are thus preempted from many of the liability concerns discussed above. If the employer's UM firm is judged, under ERISA, to have "fiduciary" responsibility (discretionary authority or control) on the plan's behalf, the firm is also exempted. The exact scope of ERISA preemption is still being clarified by the courts. Uncertainty remains.

ERISA also limits the extent of damages awarded against ERISA qualified plans. The monetary award is usually equivalent to the recovery of the plan's benefits, *not* awards for pain and suffering. Also, jury trials are not a right under ERISA regulations, while awards for the plaintiff's attorney fees are allowed. These aspects of ERISA provide a substantial disincentive to bring litigation against employer plans.

SUMMARY

The Supreme Court's interpretation of ERISA limits much litigation against MMHC entities that have UM functions. Under the HMO rubric, much more litigation is precluded by the arbitration clause in provider contracts. These clauses often bind the parties to settle any disputes through a predetermined arbitration process. Despite these protections, UM firms, employers, insurance carriers and their personnel are at risk for litigation by dissatisfied consumers and providers. This is especially the case when UM processes are not clearly defined, followed, and documented. The courts, state legislatures (in absence of national health care policies and universal health care systems), and governmental regulatory agencies are likely to make, interpret, and implement statutes and regulations concerning utilization review. Clinicians and employers should keep abreast of these developments and offer their input. Utilization management and MMHC firms surely will.

REFERENCES

Helvestine, W. A. (1989). Legal implications of utilization review. In B. H. Gray & M. J. Field (Eds.), *Controlling costs and changing patient care: The role of utilization management* (pp. 169-204). Washington, DC: Institute of Medicine National Academy Press.

Staff. (1990, October). Wickline court backtracks in Wilson, says UR firms bear liability for bad decision making. *Managed Care Law Outlook*, pp. 2-4.

Pollard, M. R., & Rinn, C. C. (1990). Employee benefit plans: New liabilities for employers. *HMO/PPO Trends*, *3* (5), 12-15.

Chapter Eight

Practice Survival
in the Era of Managed Care:
Clinical and Marketing Implications

IMPLICATIONS FOR CLINICIANS

As the number of people enrolled in HMOs increases, as self-insured employers seek new ways to manage the costs of providing mental health and substance abuse benefits, and as EAPs take on more of the features of MMHC systems, practitioners are understandably concerned about how these changes affect their practices and careers. This chapter discusses some of the most salient implications for change in clinical practice brought about by MMHC entities. It also suggests strategies that will assist the mental health professional in retaining as much control as possible of his or her professional future.

OUTPATIENT PRACTICE

Employment Opportunities

MMHC represents the corporatization of mental health services and a diminution of the "cottage industry" nature of the field. One important aspect of this corporatization is that more and more clinicians are employed directly by these MMHC firms. The exact number of therapists employed by MMHC and EAP firms is not known. The largest of these firms employ hundreds of clinicians directly. Thousands more are employed indirectly as network providers or affiliates. These numbers will grow dramatically in the coming years as MMHC continues to expand in both size and acceptance.

As this growth occurs, competition for competent staff will escalate salary and benefit packages, making MMHC and EAP settings increasingly attractive to clinicians as career opportunities. Individuals whose treatment backgrounds feature experience with interventions that are successful at promoting rapid change in patients will be especially in demand. Also in demand will be clinicians who have practice experience in both inpatient and outpatient settings, who have keen assessment and diagnostic skills, and who enjoy a treatment team milieu as a work environment. A knowledge of the workings of MMHC systems will be essential to all clinicians interested in careers in these challenging settings.*

While excellent skills are essential, of even more importance to these clinicians may be a sharing of values associated with managed care entities. "Clinicians most suited to managed care are those who receive their reward from seeing patients recover rapidly and in seeing mental health and substance abuse (benefits) extended to cover all employees," according to Nicholas A. Cummings, PhD, Chief Executive Officer of American Biodyne, Inc., a national MMHC firm based in San Francisco. A former president of the American Psychological Association, Cummings points out that therapists who are successful in managed care settings share a belief that unless managed care is successful in its mission, many employers will choose to reduce or eliminate benefit coverage altogether due to increasing costs (Personal communication, 1990).

For clinicians interested in careers in the MMHC industry, there are several types of positions in most such systems. Clinical managers in MMHC hold positions such as Executive Director or Network Manager. These are challenging positions involving much clinical and managerial skills. These individuals must have the knowledge of clinical, financial, and administrative systems necessary to manage the complexities of MMHC operations, while interfacing with employer, HMO, or insurance carrier customers. The recruitment and development of provider networks is a key task of this position.

A variety of clinical positions are found in these systems, includ-

---

*See Bistline, J. L. et al. (January 1991). "Five Critical Skills for Mental Health Counselors in Managed Health Care." *Journal of Mental Health Counseling* 13(1), 147-152.

ing challenging supervisory roles. Important aspects of supervisors' roles include facilitating training and staff development, leading clinical case staffings, monitoring the delivery of clinical services, providing customer service functions, and interacting with network providers. Supervisors in MMHC systems must have a thorough knowledge of managed care operations as well as diverse clinical skills and knowledge of community resources.

The clinical case manager is a key position in MMHC systems. In some operations this individual provides direct assessment and treatment services. In systems that heavily utilize a provider network for treatment services, the clinical case manager may serve a utilization management role, interacting with the treatment provider in developing treatment plans, providing peer consultation, and maintaining an ongoing dialogue with the provider to ensure the timely and appropriate delivery of care. At the same time, this case manager explores and evaluates the totality of applicable community resources available to the client, recommending such resources as would supplement direct treatment services. Examples include self-help and support groups, educational programs, or social services. Substantial skills for interacting with various individuals, as well as clinical acumen are essential in this role.

Another key clinical role is that of utilization management worker. The tasks and skills associated with this position parallel that of the clinical case manager. The role involves the interpretation of clinical criteria for admission to inpatient or outpatient treatment, as well as the determination of length of stay at all levels of care. Psychiatric nurses often fulfill these roles in MMHC, but other professionals such as clinical social workers, psychologists, and professional counselors as well as physicians are also involved in utilization management functions.

Besides these positions, many other evolving professional roles are found in MMHC systems. Psychiatrists and addictionologists serve in clinical and clinical managerial positions, often playing major roles in utilization and peer review, and quality assurance efforts. As MMHC and EAP systems merge, more and more specialists with experience and skills in both areas of practice will be employed in the emerging generation of products that have features of both MMHC and EAPs. Other specialty positions center upon network development, customer services, and technical sales.

Private Practice Survival Skills

While MMHC offers various employment opportunities for practitioners, it presents important implications for clinicians who choose to pursue private practice careers. Many private practitioners are understandably concerned about the changes brought about by MMHC. Some wonder if managed care may mean the demise of private therapy and counseling practices. Undoubtedly, for some this will be this case, as they are unable to accommodate the necessary changes in practice patterns or are too inefficient or ineffective to withstand the test of increased accountability and structure demanded by managed care.

Table 8-1 summarizes the changes in traditional office-based therapy that managed care has brought about, and will bring about increasingly. Some of these involve attitudinal change by practitioners, others involve changes in clinical techniques, while still others involve new marketing and strategic approaches to the business of private practice.

Attitudinal Changes

Most clinicians have been schooled to view the client as the "customer." Much clinical focus by private practitioners has been upon client service and the fostering of the client-therapist relationship to the exclusion of other influences. Managed care forces a reevaluation and modification of this attitude to include the MMHC (or EAP firm) as the customer as well, taking into consideration the overall goals and objectives of the referral source. These goals may include the return of the client to an optimal, if not maximal, state of functioning as soon as possible; the compliance with utilization review procedures; and the adequate documentation of services delivered and outcome achieved.

EAP professionals, accustomed to serving both the employer's goals and the individual client's goals, are familiar with the duality. Similarly, school social workers, psychologists, and guidance counselors are also familiar with this mindset, as are professionals employed in various agency settings.

Traditionally, client advocacy has centered upon a more narrow, individual perspective than that favored by managed care. Advocacy must be redefined to include an enlarged perspective, with a

TABLE 8-1. The Effects of Managed Care on Practice

Traditional Approaches	Emerging Approaches
Client As Customer	Client and MMHC/EAP Firms As Customers
Uni-dimensional Client Advocacy	Multi-dimensional Client Advocacy
Minimal Accountability	Increased Accountability
Minimal Focus on Time-Sensitive Treatments	Increased Focus on Time-Sensitive Treatments
Minimal Focus on Resource Management	Increased Focus on Resource Management
Retrospective Authorization for Reimbursement of Services	Pre-Authorization for Reimbursement of Services
Self-Directed Client Referrals	Other-Directed Client Referrals
Solo Practice	Group Practice
Marketing Aimed at the Public (Retail)	Marketing Aimed at MMHC and EAP Firms (Wholesale)
Less Entrepreneurial Approach	Increased Entrepreneurial Focus

view toward benefit protection and client education. Clinicians working within managed care systems "advocate" for clients by educating them about the limitations to therapy, as well as its benefits; by educating clients as to their financial responsibilities and options within the benefit plan they and their employer have purchased; and by thoroughly documenting and communicating treatment needs, goals, and progress toward such ends. Misguided efforts at client advocacy include expressing resentments toward managed care indirectly through the client. This is a nonproductive and nontherapeutic approach.

Accountability in private mental health practice has long meant accountability to client service, while meeting the minimal requirements for maintenance of licensure and professional affiliation. Accountability for efficiency and effectiveness have long been absent, unlike many other fields of endeavor.

Managed care demands much more accountability, both for efficacy and efficiency. In an era in which the insurance carrier served mostly as a passive claims payor, reimbursement for clinical services was not necessarily related to the client improvement. Since reimbursement was not outcome-related, an incentive existed to continue to see the client as long as the client felt therapy was beneficial, regardless of significant change or in the absence of it. Managed care has reversed this dynamic. MMHC seeks to select effective therapists for inclusion in its networks. It asks practitioners to set realistic treatment goals, to document progress, recommend new therapy approaches to replace ones that are not successful, and terminate therapy when goals have been achieved.

Clinical Changes

With its goal of returning clients to normal levels of functioning as quickly as possible, managed care has provided impetus to the development of new clinical innovations. Clinicians are examining how to modify a variety of approaches that are more compatible to managed care philosophies.

Prominent among these approaches are the so-called "time-sensitive," "solution-focused," or "brief" therapy strategies. A central theme of these approaches is that therapy is delivered intermittently, as needed, over the course of human development and that the least invasive treatment needed to achieve change is the most desirable one. (Table 8-2 compares and contrasts the values of practitioners utilizing these interventions with traditional therapists, as viewed by two well-known practitioners in this area.) Practitioners of these interventions believe that much therapy work can be done

TABLE 8-2. Comparative Dominant Values of the Long-Term and Short-Term Therapist (From Budman & Gurman [1983]. The practice of brief therapy. *Professional Psychology: Research and Practice, 14*, pp. 277-292)

Long-term therapist	Short-term therapist
1. Seeks change in basic character.	Prefers pragmatism, parsimony, and least radical intervention, and does not believe in notion of "cure."
2. Believes that significant psychological change is unlikely in everyday life.	Maintains an adult developmental perspective from which significant psychological change is viewed as inevitable.
3. Sees presenting problems as reflecting more basic pathology.	Emphasizes patient's strengths and resources; presenting problems are taken seriously (although not necessarily at face value).
4. Wants to "be there" as patient makes significant changes.	Accepts that many changes will occur "after therapy" and will not be observable to the therapist.
5. Sees therapy as having a "timeless" quality and is patient and willing to wait for change.	Does not accept the timelessness of some models of therapy.
6. Unconsciously recognizes the fiscal convenience of maintaining long-term patients.	Fiscal issues often muted, either by the nature of the therapist's practice or by the organizational structure for reimbursement.
7. Views psychotherapy as almost always benign and useful.	Views psychotherapy as being sometimes useful and sometimes harmful.
8. Sees patient's being in therapy as the most important part of patient's life.	Sees being in the world as more important than being in therapy.

in short periods of therapy, sometimes even one or two visits. (See Table 8-3).

TABLE 8-3. Treatment Goals Suitable for a One to Two Visit Treatment Course

1. Disabuse clients of false notion that their or their children's behavior is abnormal.
2. Confirm that a strategy (for dealing with a problem) devised by a client is a reasonable one, i.e., reassure clients that they are "on the right course."
3. Refer clients to self-help groups, bibliotherapy, or other such resources when available.
4. Acknowledge that a problem is not amenable to psychotherapy.
5. Describe a simple technique that is effective for treating a circumscribed problem.
6. Inform clients that another agency or institution is available and/or obligated to assist the client, especially when there is no cost, e.g., the school system's obligation to assess suspected learning disabilities.

Adapted from: Pekarik, Gene. *Rationale, Training, and Implementation of Time Sensitive Treatments.* Unpublished Manuscript 1990.

Research on treatment outcomes and client preferences supports the use of these strategies, even though such interventions have commonly been perceived by many clinicians as inferior to "long-term" treatment. MMHC will likely provide support for the development and acceptance of these and other innovative approaches to outpatient treatment. Much more research is needed in this area and should be aimed at guiding clinicians as to when such brief interventions are most effective.

The management of treatment resources on an aggregate level is a key task of the MMHC industry. In practice this means clinicians must develop and provide services whenever possible that are effective alternatives to more costly interventions, such as hospitalization. For example, a benefit plan may provide for a maximum of twenty outpatient visits per calendar year, yet the member may need more than one course of treatment in that period. The clinician must be sensitive to these resource limitations and design interventions accordingly. Outpatient practitioners working with managed care systems must also be sensitive to treatment resource management.

Traditionally, practitioners have become accustomed to providing services, submitting claims, having these claims retrospectively reviewed and — hopefully — paid. Managed care changes this process as well, with its focus on the preauthorization of services that it reimburses. This assures the clinician that payment will be made for services rendered. The implication of this system is that the practitioner must comply with the MMHC's authorization and utilization review procedures, providing only services authorized in advance. This system eliminates the guesswork of whether or not payors will reimburse providers for services rendered, helping clinicians have a more successful practice.

Clinical Innovation:
Prescription for Escalating Mental Health Care Costs

America's health care bill will soon exceed $750 billion, or over 12% of the gross national product. Western Europe and Japan, by contrast, spend only about 6% to 9% of their GNP on health care with little difference in outcomes.

Between 1980 and 1984 adolescent admissions to psychiatric hospitals increased 350%. At any time, as much as 25% of all hospital beds are occupied by psychiatric or substance abuse patients. During the last decade the cost of psychiatric care, fueled in large part by hospital costs, rose at twice the rate of the overall medical consumer price index. Today as much as 70% of employers' mental health benefit dollars go toward mental health related hospitalization. Rather than eliminate these benefits, employers may turn to managed mental health care specialists for solutions.

One clinical innovation is Psychiatric Home Health Care (PHHC). This service provides intensive, outpatient treatment to clients whose conditions would traditionally warrant hospitalization. Unlike partial hospitalization programs, which are often associated with psychiatric hospitals and may sometimes produce ever longer treatment episodes, these services are offered in the client's home. Clients and families are seen when needed, twenty-four hours a day, seven days a week. PHHC services teach clients how to cope and resolve problems in living and support independence. They may even provide more direct treatment hours per day, at less cost than hospital-based care. Clients who are acutely suicidal, homicidal, or are severely psychotic or manic are inappropriate for such care but may utilize such services after stabilization in a hospital setting. However, many acute clients can be treated by these intensive in-home services, averting hospitalizations. These and other clinical innovations aimed at reducing unnecessary psychiatric hospitalizations are increasingly of interest to EAP and MMHC professionals.*

The Practitioner as Entrepreneur

The managed care environment creates an atmosphere more conducive to the success of creative, entrepreneurally-oriented therapists. Such therapists will be quick to see how MMHC is influencing the business of their practices and adjust accordingly. Here are some examples of these changes.

Managed care represents the introduction of a wholesaling influence in the market for therapy and counseling services. The prevailing hypothesis among employers and other purchasers of needed treatment services is that complete freedom of choice to access treatment on the part of consumers results in unnecessary costs and that management of this process by qualified professionals is needed. The translation of this hypothesis into action means that through a single agreement between an employer and a MMHC or EAP firm tens of thousands of consumers will be directed toward a selected group of treatment providers. Self-referrals by individuals to therapists will represent diminishing volumes of clients in coming years. More the norm will be referrals directed to the practitioner by others (MMHC case managers or EAP professionals), or by the design of the client's benefit plan which provides a financial incentive to the consumer to utilize certain clinicians endorsed by the plan's managers. This endorsement (inclusion in provider networks) will, of course, be based on the practitioners' practice patterns, efficiency, and acceptance of fee discounts.

Because MMHC uses alternative fee arrangements such as fee discounting and fixed fee maximums, outpatient, office-based practitioners affiliated with MMHC system have a need to keep their

---

*For a discussion of these services and the literature concerning their effectiveness see: Pigott, H. E. (1991). "Psychiatric Home Health Care: One Prescription for Soaring Mental Health Costs." In *Driving Down Health Care Costs, Strategies & Solutions: 1991* (pp. 9.1-9.10.) New York: Panel Publishers.

operational cost as low as is feasible. An increase in managed care in the future will give momentum toward the establishment of more group practices, where overhead costs may be shared and reduced in relation to each practitioner. These arrangements may also facilitate the development of group therapies as an efficient and effective treatment modality. Group therapy is often not compatible with the reduced client volume associated with a solo practice.

Managed care holds the potential to revolutionize how practitioners have approached the marketing of their services. In the past many practitioners have become successful by analyzing their communities' needs; developing a specialization or niche to fit a particular need or needs; and publicizing the service provided through mass media advertising, promotional literature, workshops, and the cultivation of collegial referral sources. Today, practitioners, especially newcomers, must aim marketing efforts at the managed care markets in their respective communities, while recognizing that competition for the decreasing number of potential clients who have total freedom of choice concerning reimbursable treatment providers will increase.

Below are several strategies to employ in marketing to the managed care industry:

1. Assess the managed care referral sources.* They include MMHC firms (local and national), EAPs, PPOs, and self-insured employers. Determine their size and attractiveness potential.

2. Assess the special needs of this market. Potential specialty needs include services for:

• assessment services
• twenty-four-hour crisis intervention services
• substance abuse programs
• eating disorders
• marital counseling

---

*Appendix B of this book contains a current list of the nation's HMOs as compiled by InterStudy, a Minnesota-based managed care research organization. Appendix E contains a list of the nation's leading MMHC and EAP firms. PPOs are referral sources, i.e., how well are they managed, how well do they reimburse for services rendered to their members? Listings of PPOs, which may or may not include a MH/SA component, can be obtained from the American Association of Preferred Provider Organizations, whose address is in the Resource Directory.

- parenting skills
- sex therapy
- partial hospitalization services
- crisis intervention services
- in-home psychiatric interventions
- ambulatory detoxification
- specialized testing or diagnostic services, such as evaluation for attention deficit hyperactivity disorder

3. Consider developing MMHC services as a part of your practice. While the capital and expertise to fund and operate an at-risk MMHC system is beyond the scope of most practitioners, other avenues are available to enter the market as a vendor. Employee assistance programs can be offered with little capital investment, can be designed to incur marginal or no financial risk for clinical services on the vendor's behalf, and require no license in most settings. Specialized training in the EAP field is required, but is readily available through seminars and university sponsored programs. A nationally recognized credential (Certified Employee Assistance Professional) is available through the Employee Assistance Professional's Association (see the Resource Directory). This credential indicates to prospective customers that you have specialized skills in this area of practice.

Also be aware that self-insured employers, which include most of the larger employers in any community, constitute a market for the vendor of a preferred provider organization, or network. PPOs are largely unregulated and small PPOs require minimal capital to develop.

4. Recognize that MMHC firms represent an important secondary market for practitioner's services. Such secondary markets can provide a steady stream of referrals to boutique practices. For example, Acme HMO does not have a benefit for marital counseling, therefore its MMHC firm does not provide these counseling services when the assessment reveals only a V code diagnosis of marital problem (DSM-III-R Code V61.10). Yet the MMHC firm has numerous potential referrals of these clients to a clinician who specializes in this area of practice and is willing to adjust her fees in such a way that clients can purchase services themselves, outside their health care benefits plan. This may also be the case for clients

presenting other excluded diagnoses or who have requests for therapy services that are not covered within their benefit plan. Table 8-4 lists these and other suitable practice strategies.

Finally, the managed care environment will reward the creative, entrepreneurial practitioners who can efficiently manage her practice while developing innovative ways to serve clients and customers. This will mean in many instances reevaluation of what skills the practitioner community has to offer to MMHC clients and a rethinking of how to develop and package them in a manner that is compatible to managed care systems.

TABLE 8-4. Successful Strategies for Private Practice Growth in a Managed Care Environment

- Use current *Diagnostic and Statistical Manual* codes and terminology.
- Make clinical notes for each visit or interaction with the client. Use a standard format such as S.O.A.P.
- Reduce overhead costs and increase economies of scale by joining with colleagues in group practices.
- Provide patient advocacy by informing patients of their rights and responsibilities within their benefit plan.
- Become familiar with MMHC utilization review procedures, forms, and appeals processes.
- View managed care as an increasingly important market for counseling and treatment services.
- View MMHC firms as important secondary markets for referrals.
- Assess the managed care market carefully, choosing the most attractive organization(s) for network affiliation. Evaluate on the basis of financial stability, competent management, reimbursement levels, claims payment history and volume of referrals. Be aware that some firms may use your professional credibility to help market their networks. Inquire carefully about their business reputation, programmatic licensure and individual license where applicable.
- Become familiar with the benefit plan and the staff that manage its clients' care.
- Stress convenience and accessibility.
- Document clinical effectiveness and client satisfaction.
- Adopt an entrepreneurial approach.

MANAGED CARE-HOSPITAL PARTNERSHIPS: IMPLICATIONS FOR SUBSTANCE ABUSE TREATMENT

Psychiatric hospitals and substance abuse inpatient facilities were a growth industry in the late 1970s and throughout the 1980s. These institutions face an inevitable contraction in the near term, due to the fact that MMHC focuses strongly on the containment of unnecessary hospital-based care. Fewer inpatients and shorter lengths of stay are likely to be a continuing trend and source of concern to hospital-based programs and providers.

Managed care entities have produced fewer inpatient referrals with shorter lengths of stay through several strategies. First, clinical systems for outpatient care have been developed and implemented to treat very acute patients who, without such specialized care, might need hospitalization. Features to these systems include: easy access for emergent cases, intensive visits and aggressive monitoring of acute clients, special case management programs for clients at high risk for hospitalization, after-hours crisis intervention services, and alternative programming such as partial hospital services.

Once hospitalized, MMHC firms have monitored care through utilization management processes (see Chapter Six) to determine that hospital care is necessary; that no less restrictive, lower cost alternative treatment setting is available; that the patient is improving as a result of care at that level of intensity; and that appropriate discharge plans are in place well before discharge.

When ready for discharge, MMHC systems have attempted to begin clients in treatment as soon as possible, ideally the day of the hospital discharge. These and other strategies have resulted in the lower admission rates and in the shorter lengths-of-stay lamented by many hospital staff and affiliates.

The inpatient substance abuse treatment field has possibly been impacted the most by managed care. This industry, which developed the twenty-eight-day inpatient treatment program to parallel insurance reimbursement patterns, is now faced with a proliferation of alternatives favored by managed care. Intensive outpatient treatment programs and partial hospitalization (or day hospitals) in their various permutations are largely replacing the traditional, fixed length of stay, hospital-based substance abuse rehabilitation programs.

A comment in a recent issue of the *U.S. Journal of Drug and Alcohol Dependence* by alcoholism treatment consultant Terence Gorski typifies the anger toward managed care by many in the inpatient substance abuse rehabilitation community. "The system as it is discriminates against alcoholics and denies them benefits they've paid for," Gorski said about denials for inpatient rehabilitation coverage. He and many others in this industry charge that managed care clinicians are concerned only with cost reductions, not client care (Meacham, 1990). The same article went on to predict that MMHC will be a factor in even more admission decisions in the future, increasing from 45% today to 90-95% by 1993!

Private psychiatric hospitals are confronted with similar implications as managed care becomes more and more the norm. Writing in the Fall 1990 edition of *Psychiatric Hospital,* Peter Boland, a health care consultant, says that these institutions themselves are partly to blame for their dilemma. "Those in the mental health care industry—and particularly in psychiatric hospitals—have largely failed to provide employers and insurers with an adequate range of treatment service options . . . " (p. 155). Boland also noted that fewer and fewer of the purchasers of services accept the argument that quality of care should be the main reason to preserve traditional treatment patterns.

Psychiatrists with inpatient-based practices have seen managed care affect them in similar ways—fewer patients and an increased emphasis on shorter lengths of stay. Since they have the responsibility for making decisions that greatly affect the cost of services, this group has felt the impact of managed care more than other professions. Like the hospital groups, they too have actively resisted managed care, undoubtedly because of its financial impact but also on grounds of quality of care issues and managed care's perceived intrusion into the special doctor-patient relationship.

One of the reasons for the development of managed care has been the lack of widely accepted standards of treatment—ones that would guide all treating clinicians toward similar patterns of care, while still allowing the adequate exercise of professional judgement. Both the American Psychiatric Association and the American

Society of Addiction Medicine are developing such standards. In part, they hope to encourage employers and insurers to use them in administration of benefits in relation to hospitalization and other treatment issues. Meanwhile, MMHC has already tackled this controversial and difficult challenge, producing its own standards for their members. This issue of treatment standards and how they may impact inpatient care will likely be an evolving topic of controversy and debate for years to come.

Strategies

How can hospitals and hospital-based practitioners respond successfully to managed care? Although the need for substance abuse and psychiatric beds decrease as managed care becomes more widespread, the need for treatment will not. Jobs formerly based in hospital settings will follow clients to less restrictive treatment settings, such as intensive outpatient treatment programs, partial hospitalization programs, and others. Clinicians must anticipate these shifts in service delivery patterns and plan accordingly.

Just as clinical employment will follow clients from private hospitals into less restrictive treatment settings, so too may psychiatric and substance abuse beds move to other settings that can provide care at reduced costs. The use of scatter beds is one such example. Scatter beds are found in general hospitals without formal psychiatric or substance abuse treatment units. Beds, dispersed throughout the facility (or grouped together in the case of "cluster beds"), are designated for mental health or substance abuse use. When supervised by a psychiatrist or addictionologist, and cared for by a properly trained nursing staff, many clients whose lethality risk does not require a secure unit can be successfully treated in these beds (Olfsm, 1990).

The absence of treatment staffs and facilities helps to reduce the cost of these beds. Lengths of stay in such beds are shorter than in traditional, freestanding psychiatric or substance abuse hospital settings (Hendryx and Bootzin, 1986). This is due to the nature of the service provided through these settings. The physician and nursing staff provide observation, assessment, and short-term stabilization with a goal in mind of discharge to outpatient treatment. These objectives often mirror those of MMHC concerning the use of hospital resources. One strategy hospitals may employ is to deemphasize formal treatment units, instead transitioning to the use of scatter or cluster beds.

The coming decade will likely witness the demise of the traditional, twenty-eight-day inpatient substance abuse treatment program, long the bellwether of the rehab field. Research has not shown that such very expensive programs are any more effective than treatment in less restrictive settings (Miller and Hester, 1986). Yet their cost is many times more than treatment in other settings. Unless proponents of these "dinosaurs" of substance abuse rehabilitation can document their superior client outcomes vis-à-vis less restrictive interventions (thus moving away from the "quality of care" arguments) such programs face a precarious future.

The need for quality hospital-based care will not go away regardless of the extent to which managed care grows. In assessing the needs of managed care entities to develop new programs and alternative services with different clinical goals, hospital-based clinicians and administrators will use the same methods discussed earlier concerning outpatient practice. For example, clinicians are implementing crisis assessment and stabilization units in some facilities. These units have as their goal the rapid diagnosis and stabilization of acute clients in a secure environment. Treatment dispositions (i.e., transfer to a hospital-based treatment unit or discharge to a less restrictive level of care) are made after one or two days of careful evaluation and observation.

Another emerging inpatient program is the variable-length-of-stay substance abuse unit. These programs provide medically necessary inpatient detoxification, with discharge decisions based on the individual client's medical status and psycho-social features. Like the staff of assessment units, the staff of these variable-length-of-stay units share a goal of discharging the client to an outpatient based treatment program, whenever possible. Hospitals with such detoxification services coupled with intensive outpatient treatment programs or partial hospital programs will be attractive to managed care groups.

In short, a challenge for hospitals in the 1990s will be to develop partnerships with managed mental health care firms and to offer services compatible to managed care philosophies. This will present opportunities for innovative programming on the part of clinical managers in hospital settings. Hospitals may dialogue with managed care firms as in the case of other referral sources. Marketing efforts must be redefined and targeted toward these organizations. Marketing activities aimed at the shrinking pool of clients who may self-refer with complete freedom of choice in selecting a treatment setting will receive less attention, and more attention will be directed to this new and growing market. Some writers have encouraged hospital-based administrators and clinicians to go even further and develop managed care services themselves (Fry, 1990)! Fry encourages hospitals to consider marketing PPOs, HMOs, EAPs and other managed care products. A more viable option is that hospitals will develop and market their own provider networks of clinicians, with the hospital as the focus point of inpatient treatment. In this scenario, the hospital can offer employers an array of services: inpatient assessment and stabilization, variable length-of-stay detoxification, partial hospitalization, intensive outpatient substance abuse treatment, and crisis intervention and outpatient therapy through a provider network of community based practitioners.

Hospital staffs and physicians can employ several strategies to facilitate a smoother working relationship with MMHC in providing covered services to clients. These strategies are as follows:

- Learn about the values, operations, benefit plans, and goals of respective MMHC firms.
- Study the MMHC firm's level of care guidelines carefully. Train staff and physicians to ensure familiarity with how and when the firm authorizes admission or ends coverage for specific conditions.
- Offer to increase the level of interaction with MMHC staff so as to facilitate a collegial relationship; i.e., joint case staffings, training programs, inservices, quality assurance programs.
- Adopt clinical objectives and services compatible with MMHC benefit plans and coverages. These objectives include: assessment, diagnosis, short-term stabilization of acute clients, dis-

charge planning focused on a rapid transition to outpatient treatment.

• Utilize hospital/MMHC liaison personnel to work with physicians to modify their treatment patterns to focus on stabilization of acute symptoms, not long-term therapy goals. (MMHC firms frequently are disinclined to rely on these liaison workers at psychiatric and substance abuse hospitals for primary communication about client's clinical status. Some firms report that these workers are not adequately trained or do not possess the necessary clinical information. Others prefer to obtain clinical information solely from the attending physician. Utilizing these workers in this manner may be more productive for hospitals interested in receiving MMHC referrals.)

• Document clinical data thoroughly, accurately, and in a timely manner. Include information such as:

  a. specific, behavioral indicators for hospital admission or continued hospital-based treatment.
  b. specific, behavioral, short-term treatment goals that have measurements for outcome.
  c. specific indicators of progress toward treatment goals, or the lack thereof.
  d. specific estimates of length-of-stay needed to achieve the treatment goals.
  e. specific interventions and responses.

• Begin the discharge planning process upon admission. Quality MMHC firms begin planning for post-hospitalization treatment services at the time the client is admitted. Hospital staff can facilitate a better working relationship that will ensure better care by recognizing and joining this process.

• Document client outcomes. Develop a data base of information concerning the clinical outcome of services provided.

• Conduct client satisfaction research. Be able to demonstrate that clients received quality care as measured by their own reports about the facility, physician staff, nursing care, and mental health professionals.

• Do not express resentments toward MMHC through the client care or improvement. Address concerns through direct contact with MMHC staff, through professional associations, or through direct communication with the employer and insurer community.

• Learn about respective MMHC firms' appeal processes for disputed coverage decisions. Train staff about these processes. Most firms have three levels of appeal:

    a. Appeal to the review staff.

    b. Appeal to the supervising clinician or medical director.

    c. Appeal to a committee or group, less directly involved with the particular case. This appeal may involve the review of all clinical records. Another reason to be sure that hospital records are well documented.

A fourth level of appeal is via a specified arbitration process described in facility-MMHC agreements. (See Appendix A for an example of such contracts.)

It is important to learn about the MMHC firm's process for appeals concerning clients whose care may be interrupted, to the client's detriment, by a UM decision. These are known as expedited or emergent appeals and are conducted while care is still being provided rather than after discharge. It is reasonable to expect such appeals to be available within twenty-four to forty-eight hours. They should be conducted by a physician on a peer review basis. The physician should be empowered by the MMHC firm to make an immediate disposition.

Hospitals should initiate an appeal after receiving written notice that coverage has been denied. Quality MMHC operations promptly issue such notices to the facility, physician provider, and the client whenever such a decision is made. If the firm does not follow this procedure, the facility should request such a notice. Facilities benefit from written policies to assist staff in when and how to initiate such appeals. Staff should be well trained in these procedures.

• Explore alternative contracting arrangements, including per diems, bed leasing, or discounted daily rates based on referral volume.

SUMMARY

As the revolution of managed care unfolds, it brings change: new employment opportunities, dramatic impacts on treatment services, implications for new marketing strategies. It is a revolution that presents challenges, pitfalls, and opportunities for all concerned, with the question of how adequate mental health care services can be preserved for the insured population of Americans at costs that they and employers can afford.

REFERENCES

American Psychiatric Association. (1987). *Diagnostic and statistical manual of mental disorders* (3rd ed.). Washington, DC: Author.

APA initiates series of actions in managed care. (1990). *Hospital and Community Psychiatry, 37,* 1106-1111.

Bartlett, J., Prest, S., & Soper, M. (1991). *Cigna level of care guidelines.* Hartford, CT: Cigna Corporation.

Beigel, J. K., & Earle, R. H. (1990). *Successful private practice in the 1990's.* New York: Brunner/Mazel Publishers.

Bistline, J. L., Sheridan, S. M., & Winegar, N. (1991). Five critical skills for mental health counselors in managed health care. *Journal of Mental Health Counseling, 13,* 147-152.

Borenstein, D. B. (1990). Managing care: A means of rationing psychiatric treatment. *Hospital and Community Psychiatry, 41,* 1095-1098.

Budman, S. H., & Gurman, A. S. (1988). *Theory and practice of brief therapy.* New York: Guilford Press.

Budman, S. H., & Gurman, A. S. (1983). The practice of brief psychotherapy. *Professional Psychology: Research and Practice, 14,* 277-292.

Dennison, R. (1990). The impact of cost containment on psychiatric practice: Implications and options. *Psychiatric Hospital, 21,* 159-164.

De Shazer, S. (1988). *Clues: Investigating solutions in brief therapy.* New York: Norton.

Developing practice parameters: An interview with John McIntyre. (1990). *Hospital and Community Psychiatry, 41,* 1103-1105.

Dorwart, R. A. (1990). Managed mental health care: Myths and realities in the 1990's. *Hospital and Community Psychiatry, 41,* 1087-1091.

Fry, J. D. (1990). Rationale for a hospital-based managed mental health care system. *Psychiatric Hospital, 21*(4), 171-173.

Forecast 1991: Managed care. (1990, December 17). *Health Week.*

Health Insurance Association of America. *HIAA on State Health Insurance Issues.* Washington, DC. (pp. 1-3).

Hendryx, M., & Bootzin R. R. (1986). Psychiatric episodes in general hospitals without psychiatric units. *Hospital and Community Psychiatry*, *37*, 1025-1029.

Hill, L. K. (1990). The future of mental health counseling in the new era of health care. In G. Seiles (Ed.), *The mental health counselor's sourcebook* (pp. 105-138). New York: Plenum Press.

Hiraisuka, J. (1990). Brief mental health care can reduce medical bills, four-year study confirms. *NASW NEWS*, *31*, 1.

Kimball, Merit C. (1990, December 17). New year, same old song: Can health costs be controlled? *Health Week*, p. 23.

Meacham, A. (1990, December). Treatment and managed care: an uneasy mix. *U.S. Journal of Drug and Alcohol Dependence*, pp. 1, 17.

Miller, W. R., & Hester, R. K. (1986). Inpatient alcoholism treatment: Who benefits? *American Psychologist*, *41*, 794-805.

National Institute of Mental Health. (1978-1979). Provisional data on federally funded community mental health centers. Report prepared by the Survey and Reports Branch, Division of Biometry & Epidemiology. Washington, DC: U.S. Government Printing Office.

Need to develop flexible practice guidelines emphasized. (1990, November). *Clinical Psychiatry News*, p. 9.

O'Hanlon, W. H., & Weiner-Davis, M. (1989). *In Search of Solutions: A New Direction in Psychotherapy*. New York: Norton.

Olfson, M. (1990). Treatment of depressed patients in general hospitals with scatter beds, cluster beds, and psychiatric units. *Hospital and Community Psychiatry*, *41*, 1106-1111.

Patterson, D. Y. (1990). Managed care: an approach to national psychiatric treatment. *Hospital and Community Psychiatry*, *41*, 1092-1095.

Pekarik, G. Follow-up adjustment of outpatient dropouts. *American Journal of Orthopsychiatry*, *53*(3) 501-511.

Pekarik, G. (1990, January 22-24). *Rationale, Training, and Implementation of Time Sensitive Treatments*. Unpublished paper presented at the MCC Companies, Inc. Executive Director's Meeting in Scottsdale, AZ.

Reding, G. R., & Maguire, B. (1973). Nonsegregated acute psychiatric admissions to general hospitals: continuity of care within the community hospital. *New England Journal of Medicine*, *289*, 185-188.

Rodriguez, A. R. (1990, Fall). Directions in contracting for psychiatric services managed care firms. *Psychiatric Hospital*, pp. 165-170.

Straussner, S. L. A. (Ed.). (1989). *Occupational Social Work Today*. The Haworth Press. New York.

Taube, C. A., Burns, B. J., & Keesler, L. (1984). Patients of psychiatrist and psychologists in office-based practice: 1980. *American Psychologist*, *39*, 1435-1447.

Using In-patient Psychiatric Benefits Wisely. (1988). National Association of Private Psychiatric Hospitals, Washington: DC (pp. 1-12).

Wagman, J. B., & Schiff J. (1990). Managed mental health care for employees:. Roles for social workers. In S. L. A. Straussner (Ed.), *Occupational Social Work Today*. Binghamton, NY: The Haworth Press. (pp. 53-66).

Winegar, N., Bistline, J. L., & Sheridan, S. M. (in press). Combining quality and cost effectiveness: Establishing a group therapy program in a managed care setting. *Families in Society*.

Chapter Nine

Implications
for Clients and Consumers

Obviously consumers are affected by changes in the mental health care delivery system. Employers, insurers, and providers should assist consumers in understanding the nature and extent of services available to them and the role of managed care systems in them. Consumers should become aware of the nature of their mental health and substance abuse benefits at the time they select a benefit option or plan. Most employers cooperate with vendors in offering orientation programs about benefits to employees. Various intracompany communications may also be used for this purpose.

The most prominent way managed care varies from traditional benefits according to many consumers is the matter of choice. Consumers in managed care systems have less choice in selecting the type, intensity, duration, and setting for care. Choice in selecting a provider is diminished as well. In managed care systems consumers are usually not able to choose a provider from the telephone book and make an appointment. Instead their health care benefit information or card directs them to a preapproved assessor or other clinician who can provide services under the plan's coverage. In other plan designs consumers must have their first visit to a treatment provider approved by a primary care physician or a company-sponsored EAP counselor. Many MMHC plans increase access to different types of providers. While traditional plans sometimes cover only the service of psychiatrists, or psychologists, MMHC networks often include these professionals as well as clinical social workers, professional counselors, marriage and family therapists, and clinical nurse specialists.

When changing to a MMHC system from a traditional one, consumers may be faced with changing a long-standing professional relationship, in favor of starting a new one with a MMHC provider. This is a relatively common scenario, given that many employer groups are redesigning their benefit plans and that MMHC firms do not include all providers in a community in this network. Instead, they screen providers and facilities. MMHC firms select only the number of providers needed to fulfill their business needs for a particular community. Importantly, they also screen for quality of services delivered, cost-effective practice patterns, provider interest, and willingness to participate in utilization management procedures. Many providers and facilities are not members of a particular network for these reasons.

Yet another change often experienced by consumers who are new to MMHC practice is a new treatment orientation on the part of the provider. Providers in MMHC systems or networks focus on the rapid restoration of normal functioning on the part of their clients. They employ techniques that are aimed at helping clients resolve their problems as quickly as possible. They take the approach toward their clients that they may return at any time in the future for more therapy should the need arise. This approach is sometimes referred to as "intermittent" therapy, that is, recognizing that there is no "cure" to many emotional and interpersonal problems, but that they can be successfully resolved and addressed again in the future if they arise. Clients learn that "more" is not necessarily better, and that results can be achieved quickly in many instances.

Consumers also find that MMHC's approach to the use of hospital care varies from tradition. MMHC uses hospital-based care primarily to stabilize symptoms and prepare clients or families for outpatient treatment. Generally, traditional benefit plans allowed for treatment to occur in hospitals, producing lengths of stay sometimes measured in weeks. MMHC systems tend to operate in much the same manner in which physicians use medical/surgical hospitals. Only clients who require hospital care to stabilize acute symptoms, or receive treatments that are unavailable on an outpatient basis, are hospitalized. MMHC staff begin planning for outpatient treatment services when the client is admitted to a hospital.

This approach to hospital care may seem troublesome to some consumers who associate treatment for alcoholism or drug abuse with an extended hospital-based treatment program. These costly programs are often fixed at twenty-eight or thirty days in length. This length of stay was derived from the maximum amount of hospital-based care covered by traditional benefit plans. For many years the only available form of treatment for addictions, these programs have helped many people. Consumers understandably are often not aware of the literature that indicates that today's outpatient treatment programs, sometimes after brief medical detoxification in a hospital or detoxification facility, are as effective in treating addiction (Miller and Hester, 1986). Families who view such hospitalization programs as a means of gaining control over a troubled family member by removing a disruptive influence from the home environment, or who do not wish to participate in outpatient treatment, may have difficulty accepting this approach. MMHC clinicians and network providers should anticipate these concerns and be prepared to address them with their clients.

Consumers find that the client payment system in MMHC is often greatly simplified in comparison to traditional benefits. The need for filing a health care claim is reduced or eliminated. Frequently the only out-of-pocket expense is a small copayment, one that is only a fraction of the actual cost of the service.

Consumers are sometimes able to receive services at no out-of-pocket expense. Often, assessment visits in MMHC networks are at no charge to the client. An increasingly popular benefit is the employee assistance program, which provides prepaid counseling services to employees and family members at no out-of-pocket expense.

Consumers in MMHC systems are protected from unscrupulous practices by providers which would put them at financial risk. For example, MMHC agreements with providers prohibit them from charging their clients more than the allowable copayment, or from continuing to provide services not authorized by the MMHC system and then charging the client. (This may be permissible, but only with the client's knowledge and permission. See the sample Individual Provider Agreement, Section 5, in Appendix A.)

Quality of services provided are often enhanced for consumers in MMHC systems, particularly through their emphasis on clinical case management. This emphasis provides better coordination of care and increased linkage to available community resources. A case from the author's practice illustrates this fact.

Diane was a forty-two-year old homemaker whose husband had recently joined a MMHC benefit plan through his employer. Diane had become known to us through an emergency admission to a network hospital due to psychotic symptoms and out-of-control behaviors. She was quickly stabilized and began treatment at our clinic, where she was assigned a case manager. Our assessment revealed that Diane had never been in a managed care system before. She had seen seven different psychiatrists since her first psychotic episode at the age of nineteen. She had also taken various psychotropic medications from at least five nonpsychiatrist physicians, and had been treated in hospitals seven different times. On one occasion, she had been transferred to a state hospital after exhausting her insurance benefits. Diane had never had a nonpsychiatrist case manager. Neither she nor her husband had ever been involved in available community-based services. Her treatment was poorly coordinated with her primary care physician. Obviously Diane needed case management services. Our clinic provided her with these services, in addition to medication maintenance by our staff psychiatrist, and a regular support group. Diane was referred to a club house program at a local mental health center. This service gave her day needed structure and provided support for achieving therapeutic gains. Care was coordinated with her primary care physician and her husband was involved in treatment. Such case management services, providing linkage and coordination of care across various systems, are inherent to well-run MMHC systems and are often absent in traditional benefit plans.

Consumers who are entering an MMHC benefit program should be aware that transition visits are typically a feature available to new members. This means that the MMHC firm may authorize visits with the client's current provider until the client may enter the new benefit plan. If treatment is nearing completion, the MMHC firm may authorize enough care so that the client can complete treatment with the present provider, avoiding a disruptive change in therapists. If therapy is not approaching completion, visits necessary to ensure a smooth transition to a MMHC network provider may be authorized and covered by the MMHC firm. Many consumers do not always understand they may have out-of-network benefits available, though at a reduced level and with greater out-of-pocket expenses. Such benefits, when available in the employer's health care plan, allow consumers greater choice in selecting providers.

Americans seem to value the freedom of choice and resist being locked into a particular system. Consumers should be given choice in their benefit plan whenever possible. They should encourage their human resource managers and benefit managers to develop such programs. They should also be aware that with increased choice comes an inherent increase in costs. After all, maximal consumer choice in traditional benefit plans is perceived as one part of the problem of escalating mental health care costs. In practice this means that overall benefit levels, premium payments, and copayments must be adjusted and be substantially different between managed and unmanaged benefits.

Consumers should view access to quality mental health related benefits as vital and understand that most employers see these benefits as worthwhile and important. Managed care strategies used by employers are ultimately aimed at preserving these benefits by ensuring quality care at reasonable costs.

IMPORTANT MMHC FEATURES FOR CONSUMERS

- Services must be preauthorized, or there is a risk of nonpayment by the benefit plan, or payment at reduced levels with greater out-of-pocket expenses.
- Treatment services eligible for benefit coverage are aimed at a quick resolution of problems.
- Hospital-based treatment programs, especially for substance abuse, are deemphasized, since most problems may be treated on an outpatient basis with less disruption to work and academic routines and increased family participation.
- MMHC networks often provide access to different types of counseling professionals, not just psychiatrists or psychologists. However not all providers in any given community are members of a particular MMHC network.
- Transition visits with current, nonnetwork providers may be

authorized for new members who are in therapy at the time they join a managed benefit plan.

• MMHC clients are responsible for copayments to providers. They usually do not file claim forms and cannot be charged for nonauthorized services without the client's permission.

REFERENCE

Miller, W. R., & Hester, R. K. (1986). Inpatient alcoholism treatment: Who benefits? *American Psychologist, 41,* 794-805.

Chapter Ten

Critical Issues

Many important questions surround the MMHC revolution and the changes it is bringing to the way services are delivered to clients and to traditional therapist-client relationships. This chapter examines the three prominent issues: the merging EAP and MMHC functions, the question of quality in MMHC systems, and the ethical issues confronting clinicians serving managed care clients.

SERVICE MODELS: CAN MANAGED CARE AND EMPLOYEE ASSISTANCE FUNCTIONS BE MERGED?

The last five to ten years have seen a proliferation both of employee assistance and managed care programs. Many internal EAPs have taken on aspects of managed care systems or plan to, while large external EAP providers such as PPC and HAI have added managed care products to their service offerings. Meanwhile, firms more closely associated with managed care, such as MCC, have expanded their lines of EAP products. Can EAPs perform MMHC functions and can MMHC deliver services traditionally associated with EAPs?

Some point to differences in the two fields that argue against any merging of functions. The first disparity, they say, is in the scope and mission of the two services. EAPs have historically had a mission of early case finding and client advocacy, whereas MMHC has minimal focus in these areas, instead concentrating on cost savings to their customers.

They also point out differences in staffing patterns. Some MMHC professionals view EAP staff as untrained and poorly qualified for the sophisticated clinical tasks found in managed care. They say that EAP professionals are too often naive about important clinical issues that dramatically influence costs. They view EAP staff as a frequent "obstacle" to managed care, saying they attempt to confound referral decisions, dispute treatment planning, and generally favor traditional treatment approaches. Meanwhile, some EAP professionals view managed care systems and staff as "barriers" to good clinical services. They see MMHC processes as impersonal and decisions as being driven more by costs than by quality of care or concern for clients.

Others point to the commonalities between EAPs and MMHC that may argue for a merging of these systems in the future. Both share a mission of ensuring cost-effective care for their clients. Both entities are organizationally comfortable with serving two clients: the individual and the corporate customer. Both entities have long been involved with clinical case management activities, both are accustomed to screening for appropriate referral resources, and both have had as their function the identification of cost-effective providers.

It seems likely that as both systems evolve, an increase merging of functions will occur. Already most EAPs are provided by outside vendors and the largest of these firms are already providing both EAP and managed care functions and services. In some instances employers may go to one vendor to purchase insurance products, HMO services, MMHC services, and EAPs.

To accommodate these changes and compete in the marketplace of the 1990s, EAPs must be able to add three key elements to their existing services: *utilization management components*, *formalized cost-effective treatment provider networks*, and *an added treatment capacity*. The first will require the addition of new skills and technologies; the second requires only a refinement of existing functions; while the third may require changes in staffing patterns as some old style EAPs used unlicensed individuals in counseling capacities. These changes will also provide an increased need for EAP administrators with managed care experience and knowledge.

In contrast, MMHC will be challenged to develop an orientation and approach more heavily focused on prevention, case finding, and customer service in order to provide EAP services or to blend them into existing products. MMHC staff will also need to develop more EAP-specific skills and knowledge. Meeting these challenges while continuing to manage costs will be critical to MMHC entities.

The uncertainty as to if and how one of these entities will supersede and supplant the other presents a range of opportunities to many organizations and entrepreneurially oriented individuals who can provide new service models. While no perfect, hybrid model exists, two possible EAP/MMHC products are found in Tables 10-1 and 10-2. The first can be adapted to smaller practice settings, while the second requires the administrative and financial resources associated with large insurance and employee benefit companies.

TABLE 10-1. A Model EAP/MMHC Product Suitable for Delivery to Employer Accounts by Small Clinical Practices

Features

• Prevention and case finding activities

— Wellness seminars
— Educational materials
— Employee orientation

• Training and consultation

— Executive orientation
— Supervisory training
— Human resource policy consultation

• Assessment, clinical case management, and extended treatment*

— Clinical assessment and referral to community resources as appropriate (broad brush approach)
— Brief treatment component, with a session limit paralleling the average number of treatment sessions required per presentation of most clinical problems.

• Provider network, contracted and credentialed

— Outpatient services
— Inpatient facilities

• Quality assurance programs

— Monitor outcomes, client satisfaction, complaints, and assure clinical standards. Performance features in the contract can be tied to these indicators, penalizing the vendor for excess complaints, poor outcomes, and excess claims costs.

---

*Mandatory/nonmandatory options regarding accessing MH/SA benefits.

TABLE 10-2. A Model EAP/MMHC Product Suitable for Delivery to Employer Accounts by Employee Benefit Companies

Features

• Prevention and case finding activities
  – Wellness seminars
  – Educational materials
  – Employee orientation

• Training and consultation
  – Executive orientation
  – Supervisory training
  – Human resource policy consultation

• Assessment, clinical case management, and extended treatment*
  – Clinical assessment and referral to community resources as appropriate (broad brush approach).
  – Brief treatment component, with a session limit paralleling the average number of treatment sessions required per presentation of most clinical problems.

• Provider network, contracted and credentialed
  – Outpatient providers
  – Inpatient facilities

• Quality assurance programs
  – Monitor outcomes, client satisfaction, complaints, and assure clinical standards. Performance features in the contract can be tied to these indicators, penalizing the vendor for excess complaints, poor outcomes, and excess claims costs.

• Utilization management
  – Preadmission certification
  – Concurrent review

• MIS reporting
  – Utilization and trending data

Discussion

This model can be sold as an "at risk" product for MH/SA services or without risk. It utilizes local EAP/MMHC staff to provide the ongoing account service, training, consultation, assessment, UM, MH/SA treatment services, provider network management, and QA functions. MIS functions involve an interface between local and central operations. This product can be sold by sales forces to employers wanting a "friendly" MMHC product or a nontraditional looking EAP.

---

*Mandatory/nonmandatory options regarding accessing MH/SA benefits.

QUALITY OF SERVICES

MMHC systems have been frequently criticized as evidencing multiple deficits concerning the delivery of quality services, both to clients and providers. Some criticisms focus on administrative services, while others are related to clinical services and philosophies. Many are testimony to the impact of managed care on traditional service delivery systems. Common criticisms include poor management, poor claims payment services, poor provider network relations, inadequate reimbursement (or excessive discounting requested) for services rendered, confusing UM procedures, excessive paperwork, and a concern that needed care is denied or not authorized for reimbursement, and that such decisions are made by unqualified staff.

While some of these concerns have been generated by the inherent structure and accountability requirements associated with managed care, others are legitimate criticisms. Managed mental health is an emerging, growth industry. There are no "standardized" models of MMHC. Just as the lack of a national health care policy has allowed the marketplace to largely shape the health care industry, in conjunction with various regulatory bodies, so too has it shaped the MMHC field. Some MMHC firms, interested mostly in short-term gains, have promised enormous savings to employers and insurers. After garnering these immediate profits, such firms have lost accounts due to practices that do not provide adequate care or provide poor customer services.

MMHC firms that will be successful in the long term are those that make a commitment to quality service delivery to three constituent groups: (1) individual clients or patients, (2) customers, and (3) providers. This commitment to quality will be found within a larger social mission of providing needed services, preserving benefits, and managing the resources society provides for mental health and substance abuse treatment services in the private sector.

What are some indicators of quality in the MMHC field? In addition to adequate administrative expertise and the financial resources to operate these delivery systems, here are some essential features indicating a quality focus in MMHC.

Clinical Care Standards or Guides. These documents must allow flexibility for individualized care, but provide a consistent and reasonable framework for recommending treatment options and services. Toward this end, the MMHC system must be able to ensure the consistent application of such standards across operating sites. Without such standards as safeguards, important treatment choices can be overly or inappropriately influenced by financial incentives or constraints, or by the idiosyncratic views of particular clinicians or clinical managers. Clinical care standards should be viewed as ongoing processes and require regular modification as new treatments or technologies become accepted.

Client Complaint Systems. The MMHC firm should have written policies describing these processes and these must be made known to consumers. Mechanisms should be in place for both local and nonlocal resolution of complaints as quickly as possible. (Some firms have a corporate-wide customer service department in addition to local customer service staff.)

Client Satisfaction Surveys. MMHC firms should regularly monitor the level of satisfaction the consumer experiences toward the MMHC firm, as well as its individual providers and facilities.

Written Treatment Plans. MMHC firms should require adequate, written treatment plans for each client, by which treatment outcomes may be evaluated.

Level of Care Guidelines. Firms should have written guides, decision trees, and policies to be utilized in guiding clinicians in referring clients to the most appropriate level of care. Again, such guidelines can reduce the possibility that level of care decisions will be influenced by financial or other such motives. These guides should be clearly enunciated to the firm's network of providers and facilities.

Qualified, Licensed Staff. MMHC firms should employ fully credentialed staff functioning in capacities within the parameters of their respective professions.

Licensed Programs. Many MMHC firms offer treatment services directly through their own staff. These programs should be licensed, where applicable, by respective regulatory bodies.

Credentialed and Adequate Provider Networks. Individual providers or facility providers should be licensed, where applicable. The MMHC firm should have policies and procedures for credentialing all providers. Networks should be adequate to conveniently service the MMHC firm's members.

Staff Training and Development. MMHC firms should adequately provide for ongoing training of their staff and network providers.

Adequate Physician Involvement. Psychiatrists should be utilized in oversight capacities, and especially in utilization management activities and in expedited appeals processes.

Quick Claims Payment. Prompt payment of claims should be made to providers who submit timely and "clean" claims documents.

Table 10-3 summarizes these indicators of quality in these systems.

TABLE 10-3. Ten Essential Quality Indicators in MMHC Systems

- Clinical Care Standards or Guides
- Quality Assurance Programs
- Client Complaint Systems
- Client Satisfaction Surveys
- Written Treatment Plans
- Level of Care Guidelines
- Qualified, Licensed Staff
- Licensed Programs
- Credentialed and Adequate Provider Networks
- Staff Training and Development
- Adequate Physician Involvement
- Quick Claims Payment

ETHICAL ISSUES FOR PRACTITIONERS

Practice in the era of managed care presents dilemmas for many clinicians. As managed care proliferates these issues will affect more and more practitioners.

MMHC often places clinicians, long accustomed to relating to colleagues in an atmosphere of mutual respect and cooperation, in the sometimes uncomfortable position of having to say no to a peer's professional judgement or recommendation. Saying no appropriately and respectfully while maintaining successful working relationships presents a challenge, especially to the staff of MMHC firms.

Equally trained in and accustomed to saying yes to clients, clinicians involved in the MMHC field also find themselves in the difficult position of saying no to client requests. They must often interpret benefits in a manner that will not please the client. At these times the clinician may seem to the client as an impediment to the service desired. This type of reaction by clients is frequently described by those in the field as one of the most difficult aspects of practice.

Some view MMHC's insertion into traditional client-therapist relationships as an undue intrusion. They believe that the clinician's ethical responsibility toward colleagues cannot be maintained in these systems. Some critics feel that MMHC exposes clinicians to an inevitable conflict concerning the best interests of clients, given these and other reasons. They are concerned that serving in part a cost management, and in part a clinical service delivery or authorization function for the client's care, is a conflictual relationship—one to be avoided. They also point out that MMHC may provide incentive for clinicians to precipitously withdraw services from clients, or that in other ways financial incentives may overly influence clinician's decisions about care.

At the same time these clinicians must also be aware of ethical standards annunciated by several groups, that point out practitioners' responsibility to society as a whole. It is not the professional's responsibility while providing adequate care, to also help keep mental health care costs as low as possible and thus help preserve these benefits for private sector employees? This implies that counseling professionals be aware of and efficient in utilizing the most effective therapies as well as evidencing a sensitivity to managing mental health care resources.

Others point out that there is a widespread perception on the part of the payors of the private health care system in this country that financial incentives on various levels have created the need for managed care. They believe that clinicians involved in MMHC must accept the challenge of interpreting and applying ethical standards appropriately in new settings and evolving relationships. They believe this to be a valuable form of client advocacy, without which the trend toward the extension of health care benefits for the treatment of psychological or substance abuse problems may be reversed.

As the managed mental health care revolution spreads, as its processes and technologies are refined, and as it gains wider acceptance in the treatment community, these ethical questions and issues surely will confront more and more clinicians, and will bear much more discussion.

Appendix A

*MENTAL HEALTH PROVIDER AGREEMENT**

This Agreement (the "Agreement") is by and between
_____ ("MCC") and _____ ("PROVIDER").

WITNESSETH

1. Purpose

WHEREAS, MCC is a corporation engaged in providing, managing and/or arranging for mental health and substance abuse services ("MH/SA Services") to Participants of various health maintenance organizations, health service plans, preferred provider organizations, insurance, labor trusts, self-insurance and ERISA plans under agreements between MCC and the entities which fund or administer such Plans ("Health Services Agreements"); and

WHEREAS, PROVIDER is duly licensed and/or certified as required by law to practice the profession of _____ in the State or Commonwealth of _____ and wishes to provide certain MH/SA Services ("Covered Services") under the terms and conditions set forth herein to Participants; and

WHEREAS, MCC desires to contract with PROVIDER to provide Covered Services for the benefit of Participants;

NOW, THEREFORE, in consideration of the premises and mutual promises herein, the parties agree as follows:

2. Definitions

a. *Accounts* — Means an employer or other entity which has established a welfare benefit plan, and which has contracted with MCC or Payor to make available the Provider Network.

---

*This is a sample document.

b. *Coinsurance* — Means that portion of the MCC considered charge for Covered Services, calculated as a percentage of the charge of such services, which is to be paid by Participants.

c. *Copayment or Deductible* — Means a fixed dollar portion of the charge of Covered Services which is to be paid by Participants.

d. *Covered Services* — Means those PROVIDER services which are listed on Exhibit A attached hereto.

e. *Medical Management Programs* — Means the quality management, credentialling, case management and other programs ad or established by MCC.

f. *Medically Necessary* — Means services or supplies which, under the provisions of this Agreement, are: (1) necessary for the symptoms, diagnosis or treatment of the mental health or substance abuse condition; (2) provided for diagnosis or direct care and treatment of the mental health or substance abuse condition; (3) not primarily for the convenience of the Participant, the Participant's physician or another PROVIDER; and (4) the most appropriate supply or level of service which can safely be provided. For inpatient stays, this means that acute care as an inpatient is necessary due to the kind of services the Participant is receiving or the severity of the Participant's condition, and that safe and adequate care cannot be received as an outpatient or in a less intensified setting.

g. *Participant* — Means any individual, or eligible dependent of such individual, whether referred to as "Insured," "Subscriber," "Member," "Participant," "Covered Life or Individual," "Enrollee," "Dependent," or otherwise, who is eligible for Covered Services pursuant to Health Services Agreements.

h. *Participating Providers* — Means those MH/SA Service providers and other health care providers or institutions who have entered into agreements with MCC to provide Covered Services to Participants.

i. *Payor* — Means MCC, or an insurer, or health maintenance organization, or employer, or other entity which funds or administers a Plan.

j. *Plan* — Means the welfare benefit plan funded, arranged, or administered by Payor for Payor's or Account's Participants.

k. *Provider Network* — Means the network of Participating Providers established and maintained by MCC to provide Covered Services to Participants.

l. *Provider Services* — Means those mental health and substance abuse services provided by a Participating Provider and covered by a Plan.

3. Provider's Obligations

a. PROVIDER shall personally provide the Medically Necessary Covered Services listed on Exhibit A to Participants in accordance with the program(s) set forth in Exhibit(s) B of this Agreement.

b. PROVIDER will maintain sufficient facilities and personnel to provide Participants with timely access to Covered Services in accordance with the standards set forth in the Medical Management Programs.

c. PROVIDER agrees to keep valid all licenses and/or certifications which are required under federal, state or local laws for the provision of Covered Services to Participants.

d. PROVIDER agrees to fully cooperate with MCC and the Plans to resolve complaints from Participants and shall use his/her best efforts to comply with the complaint procedures established by MCC and/or each of the Plans.

e. PROVIDER represents and warrants that the information contained on his/her Provider Application, which is incorporated herein by reference, is true and accurate and he/she will notify MCC promptly of any material change in the information on such Application.

f. PROVIDER will procure and maintain adequate policies of comprehensive general liability, professional liability and other insurance, in amounts deemed appropriate by MCC based on the PROVIDER's mode of practice/specialty, necessary to insure the PROVIDER against any claim or claims for damages arising out of personal injuries or death occasioned directly or indirectly in connection with the provision of services pursuant to this Agreement. PROVIDER will submit evidence of such coverage to MCC upon request, and will notify MCC at least thirty (30) days prior to the expiration, termination or material change in the coverages listed on the Provider's Application.

g. PROVIDER will not discriminate against any Participant on the basis of source of payment, race, color, gender, sexual orientation, age, religion, national origin, handicap or health status in providing services under this Agreement.

h. PROVIDER will render Covered Services to all Participants in an appropriate, timely and cost effective manner. Further, PROVIDER agrees to furnish the services according to generally accepted medical, mental health and substance abuse practice, community standards and applicable laws and regulations. In the event PROVIDER discovers that a claim, suit, or criminal or administrative proceeding has been brought or may be brought against PROVIDER relating to the quality of services provided to Participants by PROVIDER or relating to PRO-VIDER's compliance with community standards and applicable laws and regulations, then PROVIDER shall notify MCC of such claims, suit or proceeding, within five (5) working days and MCC shall determine whether to terminate this Agreement pursuant to section 9.

i. PROVIDER will maintain the confidentiality of information contained in Participants' medical records and will only release such records: (1) in accordance with this Agreement, (2) subject to applicable laws, regulations, or orders of any court of law, or (3) with the written consent of the Participant.

j. PROVIDER will cooperate with Medical Management Programs. PRO-VIDER shall use best efforts to obtain an appropriate release and keep MCC and the primary care physician or referring physician, if different, informed of the diagnosis or prognosis of treatment provided to Participant.

k. PROVIDER agrees to participate in a Provider Network for additional Accounts of MCC or Payor or with additional Payors on the terms set forth herein. No further consent of PROVIDER shall be required for MCC to add or delete an Account or Payor.

4. Compensation

PROVIDER agrees to accept reimbursement from Payor in the amount set forth in the appropriate Exhibit(s) C and in accordance with this Agreement, its Exhibit(s) and the terms of the Participant's Plan as full payment for Covered Services rendered to such Participant. Payor shall notify PROVIDER of the Copayment, Deductible, or Coinsurance, if any, which shall be charged to the Participant pursuant to the Participant's coverage under Participant's Plan.

PROVIDER shall submit an itemized bill for Covered Services personally rendered by PROVIDER on forms acceptable to Payor within sixty (60) days from the date of Covered Services being rendered. PROVIDER shall supply any additional information reasonably requested by MCC to verify that PROVIDER rendered Covered Services and the usual charges for such services. Payor may deny payment not submitted within the sixty

(60) days from the date of Covered Services being rendered, unless PRO-VIDER can demonstrate to Payor's satisfaction that there was good cause for such delay. Payor may deny payment for services that are not Covered Services or not Medically Necessary.

5. Charges to Participants

PROVIDER agrees that it will hold harmless and will not seek reimbursement from Participants for Covered Services for which Payor is financially responsible, or for non-Covered Services for which authorization was denied by MCC, unless Participant agreed in writing prior to the delivery of the services to be billed. PROVIDER further agrees that PRO-VIDER shall only bill Participants for Copayments, Coinsurance and Deductible amounts required by the Plan, and for those non-Covered Services for which Participant's agreement has been obtained as described herein.

PROVIDER further agrees (1) this provision shall survive the termination of the Agreement for Covered Services rendered prior to its termination regardless of the cause giving rise to termination and that (2) this provision supersedes any oral or written contrary agreement heretofore entered into between PROVIDER and Participants or anyone acting on their behalf.

6. Access to Books and Records

PROVIDER will maintain medical, financial and administrative records, concerning services provided to Participants pursuant to this Agreement, in accordance with applicable Federal and state laws. MCC, its authorized representatives and duly authorized third parties, such as but not limited to governmental and regulatory agencies, will have the right to inspect, review and make copies of such records directly related to services rendered to Participants. Such review and duplication shall be allowed upon reasonable notice during regular business hours and shall be subject to all applicable laws and regulations concerning confidentiality of such data or records. This provision shall survive the termination of this Agreement.

7. Relationship of Parties

The parties to this Agreement are independent contractors. This Agreement shall not create an employer-employee partnership or a joint venture relationship between or among Payor, PROVIDER or any of their respective directors, officers, employees or other representatives. This Agreement shall not be deemed to create any rights or remedies in persons who are not parties to this Agreement except as otherwise set forth herein.

PROVIDER agrees not to allow determinations pursuant to Medical Management Programs or any other terms and conditions of this Agreement to alter or affect his/her standards of care, medical judgement or the PROVIDER-patient relationship.

Each party agrees to refrain from making disparaging statements that interfere with the contractual relationships between the other party and its existing or prospective Participants, Accounts, Participating Providers, or patients during the term of or following the termination of this Agreement.

8. Dispute Resolution Procedure

In the event any dispute shall arise with respect to the performance or interpretation of this Agreement, all matters in controversy shall be submitted to MCC for review and resolution pursuant to MCC's Medical Management Programs. If PROVIDER is not satisfied with the resolution, PROVIDER may submit the matter to MCC's President or his designee who will review the matter and may seek written statements as appropriate. The decision of MCC will be binding on MCC and PROVIDER if the resolution is accepted by PROVIDER. Neither party shall cease or diminish its performance under the Agreement pending dispute resolution.

If PROVIDER is not satisfied with such resolution and to the extent permitted by law, the matter in controversy shall be submitted either to a dispute resolution entity, or to a single arbitrator selected by the American Arbitration Association, as the parties shall agree within sixty (60) days of MCC's final decision. If the matter is submitted to arbitration, it shall be conducted in accordance with the commercial arbitration rules of the American Arbitration Association. The arbitrator shall be a person who has knowledge of and is experienced in the health care delivery field. Arbitration shall take place in _____. Both parties expressly covenant and agree to be bound by the decision of the dispute resolution entity or arbitrator as final determination of the matter in dispute. Each party shall assume its own costs, but shall share the cost of the resolution entity equally. Judgment upon the award rendered by the resolution entity may be entered in any court having jurisdiction.

9. Term and Termination

a. *Term* — The initial term of this Agreement shall begin on the Effective Date and shall continue unless terminated as set forth below.

b. This Agreement may be terminated by either party, without cause, upon ninety (90) days prior written notice to the other party.

c. Either party may terminate this Agreement for cause upon thirty (30) days written notice to the other party specifying the manner in which that party has materially breached its obligations pursuant to the Agreement. The Agreement shall terminate automatically at the expiration of such thirty (30) day period if that party has not cured its breach within such period and delivered evidence of such cure to nonbreaching party.

d. MCC may terminate this Agreement immediately upon the occurrence of any of the following: (1) PROVIDER fails to maintain any license or certification required to provide Covered Services; (2) any of PROVIDER's insurance required by this Agreement is canceled; (3) PROVIDER willfully breaches, habitually neglects or continually fails to perform professional duties; (4) PROVIDER commits or fails to commit an act which is determined by MCC to be detrimental to the reputation, operation or activities of MCC or Payor; (5) an administrative finding or judgment of professional misconduct on the part of PROVIDER or PROVIDER's Professional Staff.

e. This Agreement may be terminated without the consent of or notice to any Account, Payor, Participant, other Participating Providers or other third parties.

10. Effect of Termination

The Agreement will be of no further force or effect as of the date of termination except that:

a. PROVIDER shall continue to accept reimbursement from Payor in accordance with the terms of this Agreement and its Exhibits as payment in full for care provided to a Participant for the balance of any MH/SA Services in progress at the time of termination. For purposes of this section, the rates set forth in the appropriate Exhibit(s) C in effect at the time of termination of this Agreement shall apply. This requirement applies only to those MH/SA Services that would have been Covered Services had the Agreement not terminated. Termination of this Agreement shall in no way be construed as affecting the provider/patient relationship.

b. The parties shall cooperate to promptly resolve any outstanding financial, administrative or patient care issues upon the termination of this Agreement.

11. References to PROVIDER

PROVIDER consents to lawful references to his/her participation in Programs, Provider Network and any informational efforts initiated by MCC or any third party on behalf of MCC. Neither party will otherwise use the other party's name, symbol, trademarks or service marks without the prior written consent of that party and will cease any such use as soon as is reasonably possible upon termination of this Agreement.

12. Coordination of Benefits

a. PROVIDER will cooperate with MCC to coordinate Plan's coverage with that of other Payors or entities that have primary responsibility to pay for Covered Services in accordance with the Participant's Plan.

b. PROVIDER shall not withhold or refuse to render Covered Services to Participants nor require Participants to pay for Covered Services pending a decision about which Payor is primarily responsible for paying for such services.

c. If Plan's coverage is considered primary coverage, in accordance with Plan's Order of Benefits Determination rules, MCC or Payor shall reimburse PROVIDER in accordance with Section II.A. of the appropriate Exhibit(s) B to this Agreement.

d. If Plan's coverage is not primary, PROVIDER shall supply MCC or Payor with copies of statements from third parties related to the payment or denial of payment for Covered Services rendered to the Participant.

e. If MCC or Payor is required to coordinate Plan's benefits with the primary Payor, MCC or Payor will reimburse PROVIDER the agreed upon amount, in accordance with Section II.A. of the appropriate Exhibit(s) B to this Agreement, less the amount for which the primary Payor is responsible, and less any applicable Copayments, Deductibles or Coinsurance charges. Neither MCC nor Payor shall participate in coordination of benefits or be required to provide any reimbursement if the total received from the Primary Payor exceeds the reimbursement rates agreed to in this Agreement.

13. Miscellaneous

a. *Amendment* — This Agreement or its Exhibits may be amended by MCC upon thirty (30) days prior written notice to PROVIDER at any time during the term of the Agreement. If an amendment is not acceptable to PROVIDER, he/she may terminate this Agreement, as of the date the amendment becomes effective, by giving written notice to MCC within thirty (30) days of receipt of the amendment. Otherwise, PROVIDER will be deemed to have accepted such amendment as of its effective date.

b. *Assignment and Subcontracting* — Neither party shall assign to or contract with another party for the performance of any of its obligations under this Agreement without the prior written consent of the other party, which shall not be unreasonably withheld. However, an assignment by MCC to a parent, affiliate or subsidiary shall not constitute an assignment for purposes of this Agreement.

c. *Entire Agreement* — This Agreement, its Exhibits, and any documents incorporated by reference constitute the entire Agreement between the parties. It supersedes any prior Agreements, promises, negotiation or representations, either oral or written, relating to the subject matter of this Agreement.

d. *Governing Law* — This Agreement shall be governed by and construed under the laws of the State or Commonwealth of _____ and in accordance with applicable Federal laws and regulations.

e. *Impossibility of Performance* — Neither party shall be deemed to be in violation of this Agreement if it is prevented from performing its obligations for reasons beyond its control, including without limitations, acts of God or of the public enemy, flood or storm, strikes, or statute, rule or action or any Federal, State, or local government or agency. The parties shall make a good faith effort, however, to ensure that Participants have access to Covered Services.

f. *Non-Exclusivity* — This Agreement shall not be construed to be an exclusive Agreement between MCC and PROVIDER, nor shall it be deemed to be an Agreement requiring MCC, Participating Providers or other PROVIDERS to refer any minimum number of Participants to PROVIDER.

g. *Notice* — Any and all notices required to be given pursuant to the terms of this Agreement must be given by United States mail, postage prepaid, return receipt requested and forwarded to the addresses on the signature page. The parties may agree to substitute the service of the U. S. Postal Service with those of nationally recognized courier services that provide signed receipt of correspondence.

h. *Regulatory Approval* — This Agreement shall be deemed to be a binding letter of intent if MCC has not received any required license or certification or MCC or Payor has not received applicable regulatory approval as of the date of the execution of this Agreement. The Agreement shall become effective on and after the date MCC receives such regulatory approval. If MCC notifies PROVIDER of its inability to obtain such licensure, certification, or regulatory approval, after due diligence, both parties shall be released from any liability pursuant to this Agreement.

i. *Severability* — In the event that a provision of the Agreement is rendered invalid or unenforceable by Federal or State Statute or Regulations, or declared null and void by any court of competent jurisdiction, the remaining provisions of this Agreement will remain in full force and effect.

j. *Waiver of Breach* — Waiver of a breach of any provision of this Agreement will not be deemed a waiver of any other breach of the Agreement.

IN WITNESS WHEREOF, the parties have executed this Agreement intending to be bound on and after _____, 19____. (Effective Date)

_____

PROVIDER

NAME: _____
(Please Print)

SIGNATURE: _____

DATE: _____

MCC: _____

BY: _____
                (Please Print)

ITS: _____
                (Title)

SIGNATURE: _____

DATE: _____

Attachments:

    Exhibits: A. Covered Services
                  B-1. HMO Programs
                  B-2. PPO Programs
                  C. Compensation

EXHIBIT A
COVERED SERVICES

These services checked below shall be Covered Services. PROVIDER shall be reimbursed according to the appropriate Exhibit(s) C under the Agreement only for those Covered Services provided to a Participant in accordance with the Participant's Plan.

*Check
If
Applicable*   *Service*

_____   1. Inpatient Consultation

_____   2. Inpatient Attending Services

_____   3. Outpatient Mental Health Services (Group)

_____   4. Outpatient Mental Health Services (Individual)

_____   5. Medication Management

_____   6. Electroconvulsive Treatment

_____   7. Intensive Outpatient Substance Abuse Treatment

_____   8. Intensive Outpatient Eating Disorder Treatment

_____   9. Biofeedback

_____   10. Miscellaneous (Specify)

_____

_____

EXHIBIT B-1
HMO PROGRAM

I. PROVIDER's Responsibilities

A. *Covered Services* — Payor shall reimburse PROVIDER as described in this Exhibit for providing Covered Services to Participants in accordance with Health Services Agreements.

B. *Referrals to Other PROVIDERS* — PROVIDER will only make referrals pursuant to MCC's Medical Management Programs.

II. Reimbursement for Covered Services

A. PROVIDER will bill Payor his/her usual charges for Covered Services rendered to Participants. Payor will only reimburse PROVIDER as a Participating Provider for Covered Services which were appropriately authorized, pursuant to MCC's Medical Management Programs. Reimbursement for Covered Services provided in an emergency shall be pursuant to MCC's Medical Management Programs. PROVIDER shall receive the lesser of: (1) PROVIDER's usual and customary charges; or (2) the maximum allowable reimbursement for such services as set forth in the appropriate Exhibit(s) C ("Maximum Reimbursement Rate"); less applicable Copayment, Deductible and Coinsurance payments received from Participants, and payments from third parties through coordination of benefits as described in section 12 of the Agreement. If a Covered Service has not been assigned a Maximum Reimbursement Rate in the appropriate Exhibit(s) C, PROVIDER will be paid at an hourly rate equivalent to the hourly psychotherapy rate in the appropriate Exhibit(s) C.

B. Payor may deny all or a portion of PROVIDER's claim specifically attributable to PROVIDER's failure to comply with the requirements of MCC's Medical Management Programs.

III. Billing

A. PROVIDER will submit all statements for Covered Services directly to MCC or Payor, as designated by MCC. The statements shall include, at a minimum, the following information: (1) Participant's name, sex, date of birth and identification number; (2) the date or dates services were rendered; (3) CPT-4 codes describing those services; (4) primary and secondary DSM-III-R diagnosis number(s) (5) PROVIDER's usual and customary fee for services rendered, and (6) the authorization number and the name of the provider actually providing care.

B. PROVIDER shall bill MCC or its designee for Covered Services within sixty (60) days from the date he/she renders such services.

C. MCC will make reasonable efforts to require Payor to make payment to PROVIDER within thirty (30) days of the receipt by MCC or its designee of a properly completed bill for Covered Services. Such payment period may be extended, however, if MCC or Payor, in good faith, requires additional time to investigate whether it is responsible for such billed services.

D. PROVIDER agrees to refrain from duplicate billing within thirty (30) days after submitting a bill for Covered Services to MCC or its designee.

EXHIBIT B-2
PPO PROGRAM

I. PROVIDER's Responsibilities

A. *Covered Services* — MCC shall arrange for PROVIDER to be reimbursed by Payor as described in this Exhibit for providing Covered Services to Participants in accordance with Health Services Agreements.

B. *Referrals to Other PROVIDERS* — PROVIDER will only make referrals pursuant to MCC's Medical Management Programs.

II. Reimbursement for Covered Services

A. PROVIDER will charge his/her usual charges for Covered Services rendered to Participants. Payor will only reimburse PROVIDER as a Participating Provider for Covered Services which were appropriately authorized, pursuant to MCC's Medical Management Programs. Reimbursement for Covered Services provided in an emergency shall be pursuant to MCC's Medical Management Programs. PROVIDER shall receive the lesser of: (1) PROVIDER's usual and customary charges; or (2) the maximum allowable reimbursement for such services as set forth in the appropriate Exhibit(s) C ("Maximum Reimbursement Rate"); less applicable Copayment, Deductible and Coinsurance payments received from Participants, and payments from third parties through coordination of benefits as described in Section XIII of the Agreement. If a Covered Service has not been assigned a Maximum Reimbursement Rate in the appropriate Exhibit(s) C, PROVIDER will be paid at an hourly rate equivalent to the hourly psychotherapy rate in the appropriate Exhibit(s) C.

B. Payor may deny all or a portion of PROVIDER's claim specifically attributable to PROVIDER's failure to comply with the requirements of MCC's Medical Management Programs.

III. Billing

A. PROVIDER agrees to accept an assignment of benefits which has been submitted by a Participant.

B. PROVIDER will submit all statements for Covered Services pursuant to assignments of benefits directly to MCC or Payor, as designated by MCC. The statements shall include, at a minimum, the following information: (1) Participant's name, sex, date of birth and identification number: (2) the date or dates services were rendered; (3) CPT-4 codes describing those services; (4) primary and secondary DSM-III-R diagnosis number(s); (5) PROVIDER's usual and customary fee for services rendered; and (6) the authorization number and the name of the provider actually providing care.

C. Pursuant to assignments of benefits, PROVIDER shall submit all statements to MCC or its designee for Covered Services within sixty (60) days from the date he/she renders such services.

D. MCC will make reasonable efforts to require Payor to make payment to PROVIDER within thirty (30) days of the receipt by MCC or its designee of a properly completed bill for Covered Services. Such payment period may be extended, however, if MCC or Payor, in good faith, requires additional time to investigate whether it is responsible for such billed services.

E. PROVIDER agrees to refrain from duplicate billing within thirty (30) days after submitting a bill for Covered Services to MCC or its designee.

F. MCC will make best efforts to verify a Participant's eligibility. If it is later determined that a patient was not a Participant, PROVIDER may bill patient directly.

MENTAL HEALTH PROVIDER AGREEMENT
(Clinic)

This Agreement (the "Agreement") is by and between
_____ ("MCC") and _____ ("PROVIDER").

WITNESSETH

1. Purpose

WHEREAS, MCC is a corporation engaged in providing, managing and/or arranging for mental health and substance abuse services ("MH/SA Services") to Participants of various health maintenance organizations, health service plans, preferred provider organizations, insurance, labor trusts, self-insurance and ERISA plans under agreements between MCC and the entities which fund or administer such Plans ("Health Services Agreements"); and

WHEREAS, PROVIDER employs professional mental health and/or substance abuse staff, and other qualified health personnel and staff ("Professional Staff"); is licensed to provide mental health and/or substance abuse services under the laws of the State of _____; and is equipped with the appropriate, licensed, and duly accredited facilities ("Facilities") necessary to provide mental health and substance abuse services to Participants; and

WHEREAS, MCC desires to contract with PROVIDER to provide Covered services for the benefit of Participants;

NOW, THEREFORE, in consideration of the premises and mutual promises herein, the parties agree as follows:

2. Definitions

a. *Accounts* — Means an employer or other entity which has established a welfare benefit plan, and which has contracted with MCC or Payor to make available the Provider Network.

b. *Clinical Staff* — Those licensed or certified members of PROVIDER's Professional Staff who directly provide Covered Services to Participants.

c. *Coinsurance* — Means that portion of the MCC considered charge for Covered Services, calculated as a percentage of the charge of such services, which is to be paid by Participants.

d. *Copayment or Deductible* — Means a fixed dollar portion of the charge of Covered Services which is to be paid by Participants.

e. *Covered Services* — Means those PROVIDER services which are listed on Exhibit A attached hereto.

f. *Medical Management Programs* — Means the quality management, credentialling, case management and other programs adopted or established by MCC.

g. *Medically Necessary* — Means services or supplies which, under the provisions of this Agreement, are: (1) necessary for the symptoms, diagnosis or treatment of the mental health or substance abuse condition; (2) provided for diagnosis or direct care and treatment of the mental health or substance abuse condition; (3) not primarily for the convenience of the Participant, the Participant's physician or another PROVIDER; and (4) the most appropriate supply or level of service which can safely be provided. For inpatient stays, this means that acute care as an inpatient is necessary due to the kind of services the Participant is receiving or the severity of the Participant's condition, and that safe and adequate care cannot be received as an outpatient or in a less intensified setting.

h. *Participant* — Means any individual, or eligible dependent of such individual, whether referred to as "Insured," "Subscriber," "Member," "Participant," "Covered Life or Individual," "Enrollee," "Dependent," or otherwise, who is eligible for Covered Services pursuant to Health Services Agreements.

i. *Participating Providers* — Means those MH/SA Service providers and other health care providers or institutions who have entered into agreements with MCC to provide Covered Services to Participants.

j. *Payor* — Means MCC, or an insurer, or health maintenance organization, or employer, or other entity which funds or administers a Plan.

k. *Plan* — Means the welfare benefit plan funded, arranged, or administered by Payor for Payor's or Account's Participants.

l. *Provider Network* — Means the network of Participating Providers established and maintained by MCC to provide Covered Services to Participants.

m. *Provider Services* — Means those mental health and substance abuse services provided by a Participating Provider and covered by a Plan.

3. Provider's Obligations

a. PROVIDER shall have all of its Clinical Staff complete MCC's Provider Application and submit such additional information as MCC requests for credentialling purposes. Further PROVIDER shall submit evidence to MCC of initial and recurring licensing or certification for each member of its Clinical Staff approved by MCC for participation. MCC will notify PROVIDER regarding which Clinical Staff have been approved for participation. PROVIDER shall be reimbursed for Covered Services rendered only by Clinical Staff whose credentials have been reviewed and approved by MCC.

b. PROVIDER, through its Clinical Staff, shall provide the Medically Necessary Covered Services listed on Exhibit A to Participants in accordance with the program(s) set forth in the appropriate Exhibit(s) B of this Agreement.

c. PROVIDER will maintain sufficient facilities and personnel to provide Participants with timely access to Covered Services in accordance with the standards set forth in the Medical Management Programs.

d. PROVIDER agrees and shall require its Clinical Staff to agree to keep valid all licenses and/or certifications which are required under federal, state or local laws for the provision of Covered Services to Participants.

e. PROVIDER agrees and shall require its Clinical Staff to agree to fully cooperate with MCC and the Plans to resolve complaints from Participants and use best efforts to comply with the complaint procedures established by MCC and/or each of the Plans.

f. PROVIDER shall require its Clinical Staff to represent and warrant that the information contained on his/her Provider Application, which is incorporated herein by reference, is true and accurate. PROVIDER will notify MCC promptly of any material change in the information on such Application.

g. PROVIDER will procure and maintain adequate policies of comprehensive general liability, professional liability and other insurance, in amounts deemed appropriate by MCC based on the PROVIDER's mode of practice/specialty, necessary to insure the PROVIDER against any claim or claims for damages arising out of personal injuries or death occasioned directly or indirectly in connection with the provision of services pursuant to this Agreement. PROVIDER will submit evidence of such coverage to MCC upon request, and will notify MCC at least thirty (30) days prior to the expiration, termination or material change in the coverages.

h. PROVIDER agrees and shall require its Clinical Staff to agree not to discriminate against any Participant on the basis of source of payment, race, color, gender, sexual orientation, age, religion, national origin, handicap or health status in providing services under this Agreement.

i. PROVIDER, through its Clinical Staff, will render Covered Services to all Participants in an appropriate, timely and cost effective manner. Further, PROVIDER, through its Clinical Staff, agrees and shall require its Clinical Staff to agree to furnish the services according to generally accepted medical, mental health and substance abuse practice, community standards and applicable laws and regulations. In the event PROVIDER discovers that a claim, suit, or criminal or administrative proceeding has been brought or may be brought against PROVIDER or a member of its Clinical Staff relating to the quality of services provided to Participants by PROVIDER or a member of its Clinical Staff or relating to the compliance of PROVIDER or a member of its Clinical Staff with community standards and applicable laws and regulations, then PROVIDER shall notify MCC of such claims, suit or proceeding, within five (5) working days and MCC shall determine whether to terminate this Agreement pursuant to section 9.

j. PROVIDER agrees and shall require its Clinical Staff to agree to maintain the confidentiality of information contained in Participants' medical records and will only release such records: (1) in accordance with this Agreement, (2) subject to applicable laws, regulations, or orders of any court of law, or (3) with the written consent of the Participant.

k. PROVIDER agrees and shall require its Clinical Staff to agree to cooperate with Medical Management Programs. PROVIDER agrees and shall require its Clinical Staff to use best efforts to obtain an appropriate release and keep MCC and the primary care physician or referring physician, if different, informed of the diagnosis or prognosis of treatment provided to Participant.

l. PROVIDER agrees to participate in a Provider Network for additional Accounts of MCC or Payor or with additional Payors on the terms set forth herein. No further consent of PROVIDER shall be required for MCC to add or delete an Account or Payor.

4. Compensation

PROVIDER agrees to accept reimbursement from Payor in the amount set forth in the appropriate Exhibit(s) C and in accordance with this Agreement, its Exhibit(s) and the terms of the Participant's Plan as full payment for Covered Services rendered to such Participant. Payor shall notify PROVIDER of the Copayment, Deductible, or Coinsurance, if any, which shall be charged to the Participant pursuant to the Participant's coverage under Participant's Plan.

PROVIDER shall submit an itemized bill for Covered Services rendered by PROVIDER on forms acceptable to Payor within sixty (60) days from the date of Covered Services being rendered. PROVIDER shall supply any additional information reasonably requested by MCC to verify that PROVIDER rendered Covered Services and the usual charges for such services. Payor may deny payment not submitted within the sixty (60) days from the date of Covered Services being rendered, unless PROVIDER can demonstrate to Payor's satisfaction that there was good cause for such delay. Payor may deny payment for services that are not Covered Services or not Medically Necessary.

5. Charges to Participants

PROVIDER agrees that it will hold harmless and will not seek reimbursement from Participants for Covered Services for which Payor is financially responsible, or for non-Covered Services for which authorization was denied by MCC, unless Participant agreed in writing prior to the delivery of the services to be billed. PROVIDER further agrees that PROVIDER shall only bill Participants for Copayments, Coinsurance and Deductible amounts required by the Plan, and for those non-Covered Services for which Participant's agreement has been obtained as described herein.

PROVIDER further agrees (1) this provision shall survive the termination of the Agreement for Covered Services rendered prior to its termination regardless of the cause giving rise to termination and that (2) this provision supersedes any oral or written contrary agreement heretofore entered into between PROVIDER and Participants or anyone acting on their behalf.

6. Access to Books and Records

PROVIDER will maintain medical, financial and administrative records, concerning services provided to Participants pursuant to this Agreement, in accordance with applicable Federal and state laws. MCC, its authorized representatives and duly authorized third parties, such as but not limited to governmental and regulatory agencies, will have the right to inspect, review and make copies of such records directly related to services rendered to Participants. Such review and duplication shall be allowed upon reasonable notice during regular business hours and shall be subject to all applicable laws and regulations concerning confidentiality of such data or records. This provision shall survive the termination of this Agreement.

7. Relationship of Parties

The parties to this Agreement are independent contractors. This Agreement shall not create an employer-employee partnership or a joint venture relationship between or among Payor, PROVIDER or any of their respective directors, officers, employees or other representatives. This Agreement shall not be deemed to create any rights or remedies in persons who are not parties to this Agreement except as otherwise set forth herein.

PROVIDER agrees and shall require its Clinical Staff to agree not to allow determinations pursuant to Medical Management Programs or any other terms and conditions of this Agreement to alter or affect standards of care, medical judgement or the PROVIDER-patient relationship.

PROVIDER agrees and shall require its Clinical Staff to agree and MCC agrees to refrain from making disparaging statements that interfere with the contractual relationships between the parties and existing or prospective Participants, Accounts, Participating Providers, or patients during the term of or following the termination of this Agreement.

8. Dispute Resolution Procedure

In the event any dispute shall arise with respect to the Performance or interpretation of this Agreement, all matters in controversy shall be submitted to MCC for review and resolution pursuant to MCC's Medical Management Programs. If PROVIDER is not satisfied with the resolution, PROVIDER may submit the matter to MCC's President or his designee who will review the matter and may seek written statements as appropriate. The decision of MCC will be binding on MCC and PROVIDER if the resolution is accepted by PROVIDER. Neither party shall cease or diminish its performance under the Agreement pending dispute resolution.

If PROVIDER is not satisfied with such resolution and to the extent permitted by law, the matter in controversy shall be submitted either to a dispute resolution entity, or to a single arbitrator selected by the American Arbitration Association, as the parties shall agree within sixty (60) days of MCC's final decision. If the matter is submitted to arbitration, it shall be conducted in accordance with the commercial arbitration rules of the American Arbitration Association. The arbitrator shall be a person who has knowledge of and is experienced in the health care delivery field. Arbitration shall take place in _____. Both parties expressly covenant and agree to be bound by the decision of the dispute resolution entity or arbitrator as final determination of the matter in dispute. Each party shall assume its own costs, but shall share the cost of the resolution entity equally. Judgment upon the award rendered by the resolution entity may be entered in any court having jurisdiction.

9. Term and Termination

a. *Term* — The initial term of this Agreement shall begin on the Effective Date and shall continue unless terminated as set forth below.

b. This Agreement may be terminated by either party, without cause, upon ninety (90) days prior written notice to the other party.

c. Either party may terminate this Agreement for cause upon thirty (30) days written notice to the other party specifying the manner in which that party has materially breached its obligations pursuant to the Agreement. The Agreement shall terminate automatically at the expiration of such thirty (30) day period if that party has not cured its breach within such period and delivered evidence of such cure to nonbreaching party.

d. MCC may terminate this Agreement immediately upon the occurrence of any of the following: (1) PROVIDER or any member of its Clinical Staff fails to maintain any license or certification required to provide Covered Services; (2) any of PROVIDER's insurance required by this Agreement is canceled; (3) PROVIDER or any member of its Clinical Staff willfully breaches, habitually neglects or continually fails to perform professional duties; (4) PROVIDER or any member of its Clinical Staff commits or fails to commit an act which is determined by MCC to be detrimental to the reputation, operation or activities of MCC or Payor; (5) an administrative finding or judgment of Professional misconduct on the part of PROVIDER or PROVIDER'S Professional Staff.

e. This Agreement may be terminated without the consent of or notice to any Account, Payor, Participant, other Participating Providers or other third parties.

10. Effect of Termination

The Agreement will be of no further force or effect as of the date of termination except that:

a. PROVIDER shall continue to accept reimbursement from Payor in accordance with the terms of this Agreement and its Exhibits as payment in full for care Provided to a Participant for the balance of any MH/SA Services in progress at the time of termination. For Purposes of this section, the rates set forth in the appropriate Exhibit(s) C in effect at the time of termination of this Agreement shall apply. This requirement applies only to those MH/SA Services that would have been Covered Services had the Agreement not terminated. Termination of this Agreement shall in no way be construed as affecting the PROVIDER-Patient relationship.

b. The parties shall cooperate to Promptly resolve any outstanding financial, administrative or Patient care issues upon the termination of this Agreement.

11. References to PROVIDER

PROVIDER consents and shall require its Clinical Staff to consent to lawful references to participation in Programs, Provider Network and any informational efforts initiated by MCC or any third party on behalf of MCC. Neither party will otherwise use the other party's name, symbol, trademarks or service marks without the prior written consent of that party and will cease any such use as soon as is reasonably possible upon termination of this Agreement.

12. Coordination of Benefits

a. PROVIDER will cooperate with MCC to coordinate Plan's coverage with that of other Payors or entities that have primary responsibility to pay for Covered Services in accordance with the Participant's Plan.

b. PROVIDER shall not withhold or refuse to render Covered Services to Participants nor require Participants to pay for Covered Services pending a decision about which Payor is primarily responsible for paying for such services.

c. If Plan's coverage is considered primary coverage, in accordance with Plan's Order of Benefits Determination rules, MCC or Payor shall reimburse PROVIDER in accordance with Section II.A. of the appropriate Exhibit(s) B to this Agreement.

d. If Plan's coverage is not primary, PROVIDER shall supply MCC or Payor with copies of statements from third parties related to the payment or denial of payment for Covered Services rendered to the Participant.

e. If MCC or Payor is required to coordinate Plan's benefits with the primary Payor, MCC or Payor will reimburse PROVIDER the agreed upon amount, in accordance with Section II.A. of the appropriate Exhibit(s) B to this Agreement, less the amount for which the primary Payor is responsible, and less any applicable Copayments, Deductibles or Coinsurance charges. Neither MCC nor Payor shall participate in coordination of benefits or be required to provide any reimbursement if the total received from the Primary Payor exceeds the reimbursement rates agreed to in this Agreement.

13. Miscellaneous

a. *Amendment* — This Agreement or its Exhibits may be amended by MCC upon thirty (30) days prior written notice to PROVIDER at any time during the term of the Agreement. If an amendment is not acceptable to PROVIDER, PROVIDER may terminate this Agreement, as of the date the amendment becomes effective, by giving written notice to MCC within thirty (30) days of receipt of the amendment. Otherwise, PROVIDER will be deemed to have accepted such amendment as of its effective date.

b. *Assignment and Subcontracting* — Neither party shall assign to or contract with another party for the performance of any of its obligations under this Agreement without the prior written consent of the other party, which shall not be unreasonably withheld. However, an assignment by MCC to a parent, affiliate or subsidiary shall not constitute an assignment for purposes of this Agreement.

c. *Entire Agreement* — This Agreement, its Exhibits, and any documents incorporated by reference constitute the entire Agreement between the parties. It Supersedes any prior Agreements, promises, negotiation or representations, either oral or written, relating to the subject matter of this Agreement.

d. *Governing Law* — This Agreement shall be governed by and construed under the laws of the State or Commonwealth of _____ and in accordance with applicable Federal laws and regulations.

e. *Impossibility of Performance* — Neither party shall be deemed to be in violation of this Agreement if it is Prevented from performing its obligations for reasons beyond its control, including without limitations, acts of God or of the public enemy, flood or storm, strikes, or statute, rule or action or any Federal, State, or local government or agency. The parties shall make a good faith effort, however, to ensure that Participants have access to Covered Services.

f. *Non-Exclusivity* — This Agreement shall not be construed to be an exclusive Agreement between MCC and PROVIDER, nor shall it be deemed to be an Agreement requiring MCC, Participating Providers or other PROVIDERS to refer any minimum number of Participants to PROVIDER.

g. *Notice* — Any and all notices required to be given pursuant to the terms of this Agreement must be given by United States mail, postage prepaid, return receipt requested and forwarded to the addresses on the signature page. The parties may agree to substitute the service of the U.S. Postal Service with those of nationally recognized courier services that provide signed receipt of correspondence.

h. *Regulatory Approval* — This Agreement shall be deemed to be a binding letter of intent if MCC has not received any required license or certification or MCC or Payor has not received applicable regulatory approval as of the date of the execution of this Agreement. The Agreement shall become effective on and after the date MCC receives such regulatory approval. If MCC notifies PROVIDER of its inability to obtain such licensure, certification, or regulatory approval, after due diligence, both parties shall be released from any liability pursuant to this Agreement.

i. *Severability* — In the event that a provision of the Agreement is rendered invalid or unenforceable by Federal or State Statute or Regulations, or declared null and void by any court of competent jurisdiction, the remaining provisions of this Agreement will remain in full force and effect.

j. *Waiver of Breach* — Waiver of a breach of any provision of this Agreement will not be deemed a waiver of any other breach of the Agreement.

IN WITNESS WHEREOF, the parties have executed this Agreement intending to be bound on and after _____, 19____. (Effective Date)

_____

PROVIDER

NAME: _____
                   (Please Print)

SIGNATURE: _____

DATE: _____

MCC: _____

BY: _____
            (Please Print)

ITS: _____
(Title)

SIGNATURE: _____

DATE: _____

Attachments:

    Exhibits: A. Covered Services
                  B-1. HMO Programs
                  B-2. PPO Programs
                  C. Compensation

EXHIBIT A
COVERED SERVICES

These services checked below shall be Covered Services. PROVIDER shall be reimbursed according to the appropriate Exhibit(s) C under the Agreement only for those Covered Services provided to a Participant in accordance with the Participant's Plan.

*Check
If
Applicable*   *Service*

_____   1. Inpatient Consultation

_____   2. Inpatient Attending Services

_____   3. Outpatient Mental Health Services (Group)

_____   4. Outpatient Mental Health Services (Individual)

_____   5. Medication Management

_____   6. Electroconvulsive Treatment

_____   7. Intensive Outpatient Substance Abuse Treatment

_____   8. Intensive Outpatient Eating Disorder Treatment

_____   9. Biofeedback

_____   10. Miscellaneous (Specify)

_____

_____

EXHIBIT B-1
HMO PROGRAM

I. PROVIDER's Responsibilities

A. *Covered Services* — Payor shall reimburse PROVIDER as described in this Exhibit for providing Covered Services to Participants in accordance with Health Services Agreements.

B. *Referrals to Other PROVIDERS* — PROVIDER agrees and will require its Clinical staff to agree to only make referrals pursuant to MCC's Medical Management Programs.

II. Reimbursement for Covered Services

A. PROVIDER will bill Payor its usual charges for Covered Services rendered to Participants. Payor will only reimburse PROVIDER as a Participating Provider for Covered Services which were appropriately authorized, pursuant to MCC's Medical Management Programs. Reimbursement for Covered Services provided in an emergency shall be pursuant to MCC's Medical Management Programs. PROVIDER shall receive the lesser of: (1) PROVIDER's usual and customary charges; or (2) the maximum allowable reimbursement for such services as set forth in the appropriate Exhibit(s) C ("Maximum Reimbursement Rate"); less applicable Copayment, Deductible and Coinsurance payments received from Participants, and payments from third parties through coordination of benefits as described in section 12 of the Agreement. If a Covered Service has not been assigned a Maximum Reimbursement Rate in the appropriate Exhibit(s) C, PROVIDER will be paid at an hourly rate equivalent to the hourly psychotherapy rate in the appropriate Exhibit(s) C.

B. Payor may deny all or a portion of PROVIDER's claim specifically attributable to PROVIDER's failure to comply with the requirements of MCC's Medical Management Programs.

III. Billing

A. PROVIDER will submit all statements for Covered Services directly to MCC or Payor, as designated by MCC. The statements shall include, at a minimum, the following information: (1) Participant's name, sex, date of birth and identification number; (2) the date or dates services were rendered; (3) CPT-4 codes describing those services; (4) primary and secondary DSM-III-R diagnosis number(s); (5) PROVIDER's usual and customary fee for services rendered; and (6) the authorization number and the name of the provider actually providing care.

B. PROVIDER shall bill MCC or its designee for Covered Services within sixty (60) days from the date services are rendered.

C. MCC will make reasonable efforts to require Payor to make payment to PROVIDER within thirty (30) days of the receipt by MCC or its designee of a properly completed bill for Covered Services. Such payment period may be extended, however, if MCC or Payor, in good faith, requires additional time to investigate whether it is responsible for such billed services.

D. PROVIDER agrees to refrain from duplicate billing within thirty (30) days after submitting a bill for Covered Services to MCC or its designee.

EXHIBIT B-2
PPO PROGRAM

I. PROVIDER's Responsibilities

A. *Covered Services* — MCC shall arrange for PROVIDER to be reimbursed by Payor as described in this Exhibit for providing Covered Services to Participants in accordance with Health Services Agreements.

B. *Referrals to Other PROVIDERS* — PROVIDER agrees and will require its Clinical Staff to agree to only make referrals pursuant to MCC's Medical Management Programs.

II. Reimbursement for Covered Services

A. PROVIDER will charge its usual charges for Covered Services rendered to Participants. Payor will only reimburse PROVIDER as a Participating Provider for Covered Services which were appropriately authorized, pursuant to MCC's Medical Management Programs. Reimbursement for Covered Services provided in an emergency shall be pursuant to MCC's Medical Management Programs. PROVIDER shall receive the lesser of: (1) PROVIDER's usual and customary charges; or (2) the maximum allowable reimbursement for such services as set forth in the appropriate Exhibit(s) C ("Maximum Reimbursement Rate"); less applicable Copayment, Deductible and Coinsurance payments received from Participants, and payments from third parties through coordination of benefits as described in Section XIII of the Agreement. If a Covered Service has not been assigned a Maximum Reimbursement Rate in the appropriate Exhibit(s) C, PROVIDER will be paid at an hourly rate equivalent to the hourly psychotherapy rate in the appropriate Exhibit(s) C.

B. Payor may deny all or a portion of PROVIDER's claim specifically attributable to PROVIDER's failure to comply with the requirements of MCC's Medical Management Programs.

III. Billing

A. PROVIDER agrees to accept an assignment of benefits which has been submitted by a Participant.

B. PROVIDER will submit all statements for Covered Services pursuant to assignments of benefits directly to MCC or Payor, as designated by

MCC. The statements shall include, at a minimum, the following information: (1) Participant's name, sex, date of birth and identification number: (2) the date or dates services were rendered; (3) CPT-4 codes describing those services; (4) primary and secondary DSM-III-R diagnosis number(s); (5) PROVIDER's usual and customary fee for services rendered; and (6) the authorization number and the name of the provider actually providing care.

C. Pursuant to assignments of benefits, PROVIDER shall submit all statements to MCC or its designee for Covered Services within sixty (60) days from the date services are rendered.

D. MCC will make reasonable efforts to require Payor to make payment to PROVIDER within thirty (30) days of the receipt by MCC or its designee of a properly completed bill for Covered Services. Such payment period may be extended, however, if MCC or Payor, in good faith, requires additional time to investigate whether it is responsible for such billed services.

E. PROVIDER agrees to refrain from duplicate billing within thirty (30) days after submitting a bill for Covered Services to MCC or its designee.

F. MCC will make best efforts to verify a Participant's eligibility. If it is later determined that a patient was not a Participant, PROVIDER may bill patient directly.

INSTITUTIONAL SERVICES AGREEMENT

This Agreement (the "Agreement") is by and between
_____ ("MCC") and _____ ("PROVIDER").

WITNESSETH

1. Purpose

WHEREAS, MCC is a corporation engaged in providing, managing and/or arranging for mental health and substance abuse services ("MH/SA Services") to Participants of various health maintenance organizations, health service plans, preferred provider organizations, insurance, labor trusts, self-insurance and ERISA plans under agreements between MCC and the entities which fund or administer such Plans ("Health Services Agreements"); and

WHEREAS, PROVIDER employs professional mental health and substance abuse staff, and other qualified health personnel and staff ("Professional Staff"); is licensed to provide MH/SA Services under applicable state law; and is equipped with the appropriately licensed and duly accredited facilities ("Facilities") necessary to provide MH/SA Services to Participants; and

WHEREAS, PROVIDER wishes to provide certain MH/SA Services ("Covered Services") under the terms and conditions set forth herein to Participants; and

WHEREAS, MCC desires to contract with PROVIDER to provide Covered Services for the benefit of Participants;

NOW, THEREFORE, in consideration of the premises and mutual promises herein, the parties agree as follows:

2. Definitions

a. *Accounts* — Means an employer or other entity which has established a welfare benefit plan, and which has contracted with MCC or Payor to make available the Provider Network.

b. *Coinsurance* — Means that portion of the MCC considered charge for Covered Services, calculated as a Percentage of the charge of such services, which is to be paid by Participants.

c. *Copayment or Deductible* — Means a fixed dollar portion of the charge of Covered Services which is to be paid by Participants.

d. *Covered Services* — Means those PROVIDER services which are listed on Exhibit A attached hereto.

e. *Medical Management Programs* — Means the quality management, credentialling, case management and other programs adopted or established by MCC.

f. *Medically Necessary* — Means services or supplies which, under the provisions of this Agreement, are: (1) necessary for the symptoms, diagnosis or treatment of the mental health or substance abuse condition; (2) provided for diagnosis or direct care and treatment of the mental health or substance abuse condition; (3) not primarily for the convenience of the Participant, the Participant's physician or another PROVIDER; and (4) the most appropriate supply or level of service which can safely be provided. For inpatient stays, this means that acute care as an inpatient is necessary due to the kind of services the Participant is receiving or the severity of the Participant's condition, and that safe and adequate care cannot be received as an outpatient or in a less intensified setting.

g. *Participant* — Means any individual, or eligible dependent of such individual, whether referred to as "Insured," "Subscriber," "Member," "Participant," "Covered Life or Individual," "Enrollee," "Dependent," or otherwise, who is eligible for Covered Services pursuant to Health Services Agreements.

h. *Participating Providers* — Means those MH/SA Service providers and other health care providers or institutions who have entered into agreements with MCC to provide Covered Services to Participants.

i. *Payor* — Means MCC, or an insurer, or health maintenance organization, or employer, or other entity which funds or administers a Plan.

j. *Plan* — Means the welfare benefit plan funded, arranged, or administered by Payor for Payor's or Account's Participants.

k. *Provider Network* — Means the network of Participating Providers established and maintained by MCC to provide Covered Services to Participants.

l. *Provider Services* — Means those mental health and substance abuse services provided by a Participating Provider and covered by a Plan.

3. Provider's Obligations

a. PROVIDER shall personally provide the Medically Necessary Covered Services listed on Exhibit A to Participants in accordance with the program(s) set forth in Exhibit(s) B of this Agreement.

b. PROVIDER will maintain sufficient facilities and personnel to provide Participants with timely access to Covered Services in accordance with the standards set forth in the Medical Management Programs. PROVIDER agrees to notify MCC of any additions or reductions in services as soon as possible.

c. PROVIDER agrees to keep valid all licenses and/or certifications which are required under federal, state or local laws for the maintenance of its Facilities and Professional Staff and for the provision of Covered Services to Participants. If a hospital, PROVIDER also agrees to maintain its accreditation by the Joint Commission on Accreditation of Health Organizations relative to its Facilities and Professional Staff.

d. PROVIDER agrees to fully cooperate with MCC and the Plans to resolve complaints from Participants and shall use its best efforts to comply with the complaint procedures established by MCC and/or each of the Plans.

e. PROVIDER represents and warrants that the information contained on its Provider Application, which is incorporated herein by reference, is true and accurate and PROVIDER will notify MCC promptly of any material change in the information on such Application.

f. PROVIDER will procure and maintain general and professional liability insurance as set forth in Section 13 of this Agreement.

g. PROVIDER will not discriminate against any Participant on the basis of source of payment, race, color, gender, sexual orientation, age, religion, national origin, handicap or health status in providing services under this Agreement.

h. PROVIDER agrees that Covered Services shall be provided by qualified Professional Staff and shall be delivered to all Participants in an appropriate, timely and cost effective manner. PROVIDER agrees to furnish the services according to generally accepted medical, mental health and substance abuse practice, community standards and applicable laws and regulations.

   PROVIDER agrees to provide Professional Staff with ongoing training and supervision according to generally accepted medical, mental health and substance abuse practice. PROVIDER shall furnish a summary of such training and supervision efforts upon request by MCC.

In the event PROVIDER discovers that a claim, suit, or criminal or administrative proceeding has been brought or may be brought against PROVIDER relating to the quality of services provided to Participants by PROVIDER or relating to PROVIDER's compliance with community standards and applicable laws and regulations, then PROVIDER shall notify MCC of such claims, suit or proceeding, within five (5) working days and MCC shall determine whether to terminate this Agreement pursuant to section 9.

i. PROVIDER will cooperate with Medical Management Programs. PROVIDER shall use best efforts to obtain an appropriate release and keep MCC and the primary care physician or referring physician, if different, informed of the diagnosis or prognosis of treatment provided to Participant.

j. PROVIDER will permit representatives designated by MCC to visit hospitalized Participants and will provide information reasonably necessary to conduct Medical Management Programs in accordance with PROVIDER policies and procedures governing such activity. PROVIDER further agrees that MCC's utilization review coordinators may call designated representatives of PROVIDER for reports concerning the status of Participants receiving inpatient services from PROVIDER subject to Section 6 of this Agreement.

k. PROVIDER agrees to participate in a Provider Network for additional Accounts of MCC or Payor or with additional Payors on the terms set forth herein. No further consent of PROVIDER shall be required for MCC to add or delete an Account or Payor.

4. Compensation

PROVIDER agrees to accept reimbursement from Payor in the amount set forth in the appropriate Exhibit(s) C and in accordance with this Agreement, its Exhibit(s) and the terms of the Participant's Plan as full payment for Covered Services rendered to such Participant. Payor shall notify PROVIDER of the Copayment, Deductible, or Coinsurance, if any, which shall be charged to the Participant pursuant to the Participant's coverage under Participant's Plan.

PROVIDER shall submit an itemized bill for Covered Services rendered by PROVIDER on forms acceptable to Payor within sixty (60) days from the date of Covered Services being rendered. PROVIDER shall supply any additional information reasonably requested by MCC to verify that PROVIDER rendered Covered Services and the usual charges for such services. Payor may deny payment not submitted within the sixty (60) days from the date of Covered Services being rendered, unless PROVIDER can demonstrate to Payor's satisfaction that there was good cause for such delay. Payor may deny payment for services that are not Covered Services or not Medically Necessary.

5. Charges to Participants

PROVIDER agrees that it will hold harmless and will not seek reimbursement from Participants for Covered Services for which Payor is financially responsible, or for non-Covered Services for which authorization was denied by MCC, unless Participant agreed in writing prior to the delivery of the services to be billed. PROVIDER further agrees that PROVIDER shall only bill Participants for Copayments, Coinsurance and Deductible amounts required by the Plan, and for those non-Covered Services for which Participant's agreement has been obtained as described herein.

PROVIDER further agrees (1) this provision shall survive the termination of the Agreement for Covered Services rendered prior to its termination regardless of the cause giving rise to termination and that (2) this provision supersedes any oral or written contrary agreement heretofore entered into between PROVIDER and Participants or anyone acting on their behalf.

6. Access to and Confidentiality of Books and Records

PROVIDER will maintain medical, financial and administrative records, concerning services provided to Participants pursuant to this Agreement, in accordance with applicable Federal and state laws, JCAHO guidelines and generally accepted business practice. MCC, its authorized representatives and duly authorized third parties, such as but not limited to governmental and regulatory agencies, will have the right to inspect, review and make copies of such records directly related to services rendered to Participants. Such review and duplication shall be allowed upon reasonable notice during regular business hours and shall be subject to all applicable laws and regulations concerning confidentiality of such data or records. This provision shall survive the termination of this Agreement.

PROVIDER will maintain the confidentiality of information contained in Participants' medical records and will only release such records: (1) in accordance with this Agreement, (2) subject to applicable laws, regulations, or orders of any court of law, or (3) with the written consent of the Participant. This section will not be construed to prevent the PROVIDER from releasing information which it has taken from or based on such records to organizations or individuals taking part in research, experimental, education or similar programs, if no identification of the Participant is made in the released information.

7. Relationship of Parties

The parties to this Agreement are independent contractors. This Agreement shall not create an employer-employee, partnership or a joint venture relationship between or among Payor, PROVIDER or any of their respective directors, officers, employees or other representatives. This Agreement shall not be deemed to create any rights or remedies in persons who are not parties to this Agreement except as otherwise set forth herein.

PROVIDER agrees not to allow determinations pursuant to Medical Management Programs or any other terms and conditions of this Agreement to alter or affect its standards of care, medical judgement or the PROVIDER-patient relationship.

Each party agrees to refrain from making disparaging statements that interfere with the contractual relationships between the other party and its existing or prospective Participants, Accounts, Participating Providers, or patients during the term of or following the termination of this Agreement.

8. Dispute Resolution Procedure

In the event any dispute shall arise with respect to the performance or interpretation of this Agreement, all matters in controversy shall be submitted to MCC for review and resolution pursuant to MCC's Medical Management Programs. If PROVIDER is not satisfied with the resolution, PROVIDER may submit the matter to MCC's President or his designee who will review the matter and may seek written statements as appropriate. The decision of MCC will be binding on MCC and PROVIDER if the resolution is accepted by PROVIDER. Neither party shall cease or diminish its performance under the Agreement pending dispute resolution.

If PROVIDER is not satisfied with such resolution and to the extent permitted by law, the matter in controversy shall be submitted either to a dispute resolution entity, or to a single arbitrator selected by the American

Arbitration Association, as the parties shall agree within sixty (60) days of MCC's final decision. If the matter is submitted to arbitration, it shall be conducted in accordance with the commercial arbitration rules of the American Arbitration Association. The arbitrator shall be a person who has knowledge of and is experienced in the health care delivery field. Arbitration shall take place in _____. Both parties expressly covenant and agree to be bound by the decision of the dispute resolution entity or arbitrator as final determination of the matter in dispute. Each party shall assume its own costs, but shall share the cost of the resolution entity equally. Judgment upon the award rendered by the resolution entity may be entered in any court having jurisdiction.

9. Term and Termination

a. *Term* — The initial term of this Agreement shall begin on the Effective Date and shall continue unless terminated as set forth below.

b. This Agreement may be terminated by either party, without cause, upon ninety (90) days prior written notice to the other party.

c. Either party may terminate this Agreement for cause upon thirty (30) days written notice to the other party specifying the manner in which that party has materially breached its obligations pursuant to the Agreement. The Agreement shall terminate automatically at the expiration of such thirty (30) day period if that party has not cured its breach within such period and delivered evidence of such cure to nonbreaching party.

d. MCC may terminate this Agreement immediately upon the occurrence of any of the following: (1) PROVIDER fails to maintain any license or certification required to provide Covered Services; (2) any of PROVIDER's insurance required by this Agreement is canceled; (3) PROVIDER willfully breaches, habitually neglects or continually fails to perform professional duties; (4) PROVIDER commits or fails to commit an act which is determined by MCC to be detrimental to the reputation, operation or activities of MCC or Payor; (5) an administrative finding or judgment of professional misconduct on the part of PROVIDER or PROVIDER's Professional Staff.

e. This Agreement may be terminated without the consent of or notice to any Account, Payor, Participant, other Participating Providers or other third parties.

10. Effect of Termination

The Agreement will be of no further force or effect as of the date of termination except that:

a. PROVIDER shall continue to accept reimbursement from Payor in accordance with the terms of this Agreement and its Exhibits as payment in full for care provided to a Participant for the balance of any MH/SA Services in progress at the time of termination. For purposes of this section, the rates set forth in the appropriate Exhibit(s) C in effect at the time of termination of this Agreement shall apply. This requirement applies only to those MH/SA Services that would have been Covered Services had the Agreement not terminated. Termination of this Agreement shall in no way be construed as affecting the provider/patient relationship.

b. The parties shall cooperate to promptly resolve any outstanding financial, administrative or patient care issues upon the termination of this Agreement.

11. References to PROVIDER

PROVIDER consents to lawful references to his/her participation in Programs, Provider Network and any informational efforts initiated by MCC or any third party on behalf of MCC. Neither party will otherwise use the other party's name, symbol, trademarks or service marks without the prior written consent of that party and will cease any such use as soon as is reasonably possible upon termination of this Agreement.

12. Coordination of Benefits

a. PROVIDER will cooperate with MCC to coordinate Plan's coverage with that of other Payors or entities that have primary responsibility to pay for Covered Services in accordance with the Participant's Plan.

b. PROVIDER shall not withhold or refuse to render Covered Services to Participants nor require Participants to pay for Covered Services pending a decision about which Payor is primarily responsible for paying for such services.

c. If Plan's coverage is considered primary coverage, in accordance with Plan's Order of Benefits Determination rules, MCC or Payor shall reimburse PROVIDER in accordance with Section II.A. of the appropriate Exhibit(s) B to this Agreement.

d. If Plan's coverage is not primary, PROVIDER shall supply MCC or Payor with copies of statements from third parties related to the payment or denial of payment for Covered Services rendered to the Participant.

e. If MCC or Payor is required to coordinate Plan's benefits with the primary Payor, MCC or Payor will reimburse PROVIDER the agreed upon amount, in accordance with Section II.A. of the appropriate Exhibit(s) B to this Agreement, less the amount for which the primary Payor is responsible, and less any applicable Copayments, Deductibles or Coinsurance charges. Neither MCC nor Payor shall participate in coordination of benefits or be required to provide any reimbursement if the total received from the Primary Payor exceeds the reimbursement rates agreed to in this Agreement.

13. Insurance and Indemnification

During the term of this Agreement PROVIDER will procure and maintain adequate policies of comprehensive general liability, professional liability or self-insurance, in amounts deemed appropriate by MCC based on the PROVIDER's mode of practice/specialty, necessary to insure PROVIDER against any claim or claims for damages arising out of personal injuries or death occasioned directly or indirectly in connection with the provision of services pursuant to this Agreement. PROVIDER will submit evidence of such coverage to MCC upon request, and will notify MCC with at least thirty (30) days written notice to MCC of any material change in or termination of such coverage. Neither party shall be liable for any loss, expense, injury, claim, demand, judgment or attorney's fees arising out of any action or failure to act by the other party, its directors, officers, employees, agents or representatives, while acting within the scope of their employment. The responsible party shall indemnify and hold the other party harmless against any and all liability and expenses arising from such claims, actions or judgments.

14. Miscellaneous

a. *Amendment* — This Agreement or its Exhibits may be amended by MCC upon thirty (30) days prior written notice to PROVIDER at any time during the term of the Agreement. If an amendment is not acceptable to PROVIDER, he/she may terminate this Agreement, as of the date the amendment becomes effective, by giving written notice to MCC within thirty (30) days of receipt of the amendment. Otherwise, PROVIDER will be deemed to have accepted such amendment as of its effective date.

b. *Assignment and Subcontracting* — Neither party shall assign to or contract with another party for the performance of any of its obligations under this Agreement without the prior written consent of the other party, which shall not be unreasonably withheld. However, an assignment by MCC to a parent, affiliate or subsidiary shall not constitute an assignment for purposes of this Agreement.

c. *Entire Agreement* — This Agreement, its Exhibits, and any documents incorporated by reference constitute the entire Agreement between the parties. It supersedes any prior Agreements, promises, negotiation or representations, either oral or written, relating to the subject matter of this Agreement.

d. *Governing Law* — This Agreement shall be governed by and construed under the laws of the State or Commonwealth of _____ and in accordance with applicable Federal laws and regulations.

e. *Impossibility of Performance* — Neither party shall be deemed to be in violation of this Agreement if it is prevented from performing its obligations for reasons beyond its control, including without limitations, acts of God or of the public enemy, flood or storm, strikes, or statute, rule or action or any Federal, State, or local government or agency. The parties shall make a good faith effort, however, to ensure that Participants have access to Covered Services.

f. *Non-Exclusivity* — This Agreement shall not be construed to be an exclusive Agreement between MCC and PROVIDER, nor shall it be deemed to be an Agreement requiring MCC, Participating Providers or other PROVIDERS to refer any minimum number of Participants to PROVIDER.

g. *Notice* — Any and all notices required to be given pursuant to the term's of this Agreement must be given by United States mail, postage prepaid, return receipt requested and forwarded to the addresses on the signature page. The parties may agree to substitute the service of the U.S. Postal Service with those of nationally recognized courier services that provide signed receipt of correspondence.

h. *Regulatory Approval* — This Agreement shall be deemed to be a binding letter of intent if MCC has not received any required license or certification or MCC or Payor has not received applicable regulatory approval as of the date of the execution of this Agreement. The Agreement shall become effective on and after the date MCC receives such regulatory approval. If MCC notifies PROVIDER of its inability to obtain such licensure, certification, or regulatory approval, after due diligence, both parties shall be released from any liability pursuant to this Agreement.

i. *Severability* — In the event that a provision of the Agreement is rendered invalid or unenforceable by Federal or State Statute or Regulations, or declared null and void by any court of competent jurisdiction, the remaining provisions of this Agreement will remain in full force and effect.

j. *Waiver of Breach* — Waiver of a breach of any provision of this Agreement will not be deemed a waiver of any other breach of the Agreement.

IN WITNESS WHEREOF, the parties have executed this Agreement intending to be bound on and after _____, 19____. (Effective Date)

PROVIDER

NAME: _____
                                    (Please Print)

SIGNATURE: _____

DATE: _____

MCC: _____

BY: _____
(Please Print)

ITS: _____
(Title)

SIGNATURE: _____

DATE: _____

Attachments:

    Exhibits: A. Covered Services
                B-1. HMO Programs
                B-2. PPO Programs
                C. Compensation

EXHIBIT A
COVERED SERVICES

These services checked below shall be Covered Services. PROVIDER shall be reimbursed according to Exhibit C under the Agreement only for those Covered Services provided to a Participant in accordance with the Participant's Plan.

*Check
If
Applicable*   *Service*

_____   1. Inpatient Mental Health Services
                 (Adult) (Open Unit)

_____   2. Inpatient Mental Health Services
                 (Adult) (Closed Unit)

_____   3. Inpatient Mental Health Services
                 (Adolescent) (Open Unit)

_____   4. Inpatient Mental Health Services
                 (Adolescent) (Closed Unit)

_____   5. Inpatient Mental Health Services
                 (Child)

_____   6. Partial Hospital Mental Health Services
                 (Adult)

_____   7. Partial Hospital Mental Health Services
                 (Adolescent)

_____   8. Outpatient Mental Health Services
                 (Group)

_____   9. Outpatient Mental Health Services
                 (Individual)

_____   10. Inpatient Attending Services

_____   11. Anesthesiology Services

_____   12. Ancillary Services Not Otherwise Included

_____   13. Emergency Room and/or Urgent Care
                 Unit Services

_____ 14. Inpatient Detoxification Services
(Adult)

_____ 15. Inpatient Detoxification Services
(Adolescent)

_____ 16. Inpatient Substance Abuse Rehabilitation
(Adult)

_____ 17. Inpatient Substance Abuse Rehabilitation
(Adolescent)

_____ 18. Intensive Outpatient Substance Abuse
Services (Adult)

_____ 19. Intensive Outpatient Substance Abuse
Services (Adolescent)

_____ 20. Inpatient Eating Disorder Rehabilitation
Services (Variable Length of Stay)

_____ 21. Intensive Outpatient Eating Disorder
Treatment Services

_____ 22. Treatment of nuclear family members
and/or significant other of substance
abusing patients

_____ 23. Miscellaneous (Specify)

_____

_____

EXHIBIT B-1
HMO PROGRAM

I. PROVIDER's Responsibilities

A. *Covered Services* — Payor shall reimburse PROVIDER as described in this Exhibit for Providing Covered Services to Participants in accordance with Health Services Agreements.

B. *Referrals to Other PROVIDERS* — PROVIDER will only make referrals pursuant to MCC's Medical Management Programs.

II. Reimbursement for Covered Services

A. PROVIDER will bill Payor its usual charges for Covered Services rendered to Participants. Payor will only reimburse PROVIDER as a Participating Provider for Covered Services which were appropriately authorized, pursuant to MCC's Medical Management Programs. Reimbursement for Covered Services Provided in an emergency shall be pursuant to MCC's Medical Management Programs. PROVIDER shall receive the lesser of: (1) PROVIDER'S usual and customary charges; or (2) the maximum allowable reimbursement for such services as set forth in the appropriate Exhibit(s) C ("Maximum Reimbursement Rate"); less applicable Copayment, Deductible and Coinsurance payments received from Participants, and payments from third parties through coordination of benefits as described in Section 12 of the Agreement. If a Covered Service has not been assigned a Maximum Reimbursement Rate in the appropriate Exhibit(s) C, PROVIDER will receive ____% of its billed charges subject to a standard reasonable and customary screening.

B. Payor may deny all or a portion of PROVIDER's claim specifically attributable to PROVIDER's failure to comply with the requirements of MCC's Medical Management Programs.

III. Billing

A. PROVIDER will submit all statements for Covered Services directly to MCC or Payor, as designated by MCC. Payor shall have the right to require that all statements be on form UB82 or HFCA 1500 or other similar form. The statements shall include, at a minimum, the following information: (1) Participant's name, sex, date of birth and identification number; (2) the date or dates services were rendered; (3) CPT-4 codes describing those services; (4) primary and secondary DSM-III-R diagnosis number(s); (5) PROVIDER's usual and customary fee for services rendered; and (6) the authorization number and the name of the Provider actually providing care.

B. PROVIDER shall bill MCC or its designee for Covered Services within sixty (60) days from the date PROVIDER renders such services.

C. MCC will make reasonable efforts to require Payor to make payment to PROVIDER within thirty (30) days of the receipt by MCC or its designee of a properly completed bill for Covered Services. Such payment period may be extended, however, if MCC or Payor, in good faith, requires additional time to investigate whether it is responsible for such billed services.

D. PROVIDER agrees to refrain from duplicate billing within thirty (30) days after submitting a bill for Covered Services to MCC or its designee.

EXHIBIT B-2
PPO PROGRAM

I. PROVIDER's Responsibilities

A. *Covered Services* — MCC shall arrange for PROVIDER to be reimbursed by Payor as described in this Exhibit for providing Covered
Services to Participants in accordance with Health Services Agreements.

B. *Referrals to Other PROVIDERS* — PROVIDER will only make referrals pursuant to MCC's Medical Management Programs.

II. Reimbursement for Covered Services

A. PROVIDER will charge its usual charges for Covered Services rendered to Participants. Payor will only reimburse PROVIDER as a Participating Provider for Covered Services which were appropriately authorized, pursuant to MCC's Medical Management Programs.
Reimbursement for Covered Services provided in an emergency shall
be pursuant to MCC's Medical Management Programs. PROVIDER
shall receive the lesser of: (1) PROVIDER's usual and customary
charges; or (2) the maximum allowable reimbursement for such services as set forth in the appropriate Exhibit(s) C ("Maximum Reimbursement Rate"); less applicable Copayment, Deductible and Coinsurance payments received from Participants, and payments from third
parties through coordination of benefits as described in Section 12 of
the Agreement. If a Covered Service has not been assigned a Maximum Reimbursement Rate in the appropriate Exhibit(s) C, PRO-
VIDER will receive ____% of its charges subject to a standard reasonable and customary screening.

B. Payor may deny all or a portion of PROVIDER's claim specifically
attributable to PROVIDER's failure to comply with the requirements
of MCC's Medical Management Programs.

III. Billing

A. PROVIDER agrees to accept an assignment of benefits which has been
submitted by a Participant.

B. PROVIDER will submit all statements for Covered Services pursuant
to assignments of benefits directly to MCC or Payor, as designated by
MCC. Payor shall have the right to require that all statements be on

form UB82 or HFCA 1500 or other similar form. The statements shall include, at a minimum, the following information: (1) Participant's name, sex, date of birth and identification number: (2) the date or dates services were rendered; (3) CPT-4 codes describing those services; (4) primary and secondary DSM-III-R diagnosis number(s); (5) PRO-VIDER's usual and customary fee for services rendered; and (6) the authorization number and the name of the provider actually providing care.

C. Pursuant to assignments of benefits, PROVIDER shall submit all statements to MCC or its designee for Covered Services within sixty (60) days from the date PROVIDER renders such services.

D. MCC will make reasonable efforts to require Payor to make payment to PROVIDER within thirty (30) days of the receipt by MCC or its designee of a properly completed bill for Covered Services. Such payment period may be extended, however, if MCC or Payor, in good faith, requires additional time to investigate whether it is responsible for such billed services.

E. PROVIDER agrees to refrain from duplicate billing within thirty (30) days after submitting a bill for Covered Services to MCC or its designee.

F. MCC will make best efforts to verify a Participant's eligibility. If it is later determined that a patient was not a Participant, PROVIDER may bill patient directly.

Appendix B

1991 InterStudy HMO listing
(by state)

As of 07/01/90

STATE HMO Metro Location Plan Name [Headquarters City]	Pure Members	Open-ended Members	Model Type	Plan Age	Profit Status	Qual Status
ALABAMA						
Birmingham, AL						
Complete Health	95,518		IPA	4	P	FQ
Health Advantage Plans, Inc. [Fairfield]	2,504		Group	3	P	NFQ
Health Maintenance Group of Birmingham	8,400		Group	12	NP	NFQ
HMO - Mobile, Inc. [Mobile]	7,506		IPA	5	P	NFQ
PARTNERS Health Plan of AL - Aetna	32,012		IPA	3	P	NFQ
Southeast Health Plan of Alabama, Inc.	43,000		IPA	5	P	NFQ
Mobile, AL						
Prime Health	25,639		Staff	5	NP	FQ
Non-Metropolitan						
West Alabama Health Services [Eutaw]	2,600		Staff	3	NP	NFQ

246

ARIZONA

Phoenix, AZ

Arizona Health Plan	12,918	1,387	IPA	3	P	NFQ
CIGNA Healthplan of Arizona - Phoenix	116,556	3,993	Mixed[r]	17	P	FQ
FHP, Inc. [Tempe]	72,968		IPA	3	P	FQ
Health Care Network of Arizona, Inc.	7,847		IPA	4	P	NFQ
HMO Arizona	30,000		IPA	2	NP	NFQ
Humana Health Plan, Inc.	16,731[a]		IPA	5	P	FQ
Lincoln National Health Plan, Inc.	2,918		IPA	6	P	FQ
The Samaritan Health Plan, Inc.	34,000		IPA	3	P	NFQ

Tucson, AZ

CIGNA Healthplan of Arizona - Tucson	14,894[a]	601	Mixed[r]	9	P	FQ
Health Horizons, Inc.	7,204		IPA	3	P	NFQ
Intergroup Prepaid Health Services of AZ	197,500		Network	8	P	FQ
PARTNERS Health Plan of Arizona - Aetna	50,482		IPA	3	P	NFQ
University Physicians HMO, Inc.	10,900[b]		Group	2	NP	FQ

As of 07/01/90

STATE HMO Metro Location Plan Name [Headquarters City]	Pure Members	Open-ended Members	Model Type	Plan Age	Profit Status	Qual Status
ARKANSAS						
Little Rock-North Little Rock, AR						
American HMO	17,236	922	Network	4	P	NFQ
Health Advantage	17,627		IPA	3	P	NFQ
HMO Arkansas	17,829		IPA	4	P	FQ
Non-Metropolitan						
United Health Care [Bull Shoals]	0	850	Staff	4	P	NFQ
CALIFORNIA						
Anaheim-Santa Ana, CA						
PacifiCare of California [Cypress]	474,472		Network	11	P	FQ
The Health Plan of America [Orange]	107,390		IPA	9	NP	FQ
Fresno, CA						
ValuCare	33,817		IPA	4	P	FQ

Los Angeles-Long Beach, CA

AmeriMed [Pasadena]	48,000		Network	17	P	NFQ
CaliforniaCare [Van Nuys]	260,877[b]		Network	3	NP	NFQ
CareAmerica Health Plans [Chatsworth]	117,745	11,400	IPA	4	P	NFQ
CIGNA Healthplan, Inc. [Glendale]	88,305	1,114	IPA	3	P	FQ
Community Health Plan	9,886		Staff	6	NP	FQ
FHP, Inc./California [Fountain Valley]	301,649		Mixed[f]	29	P	FQ
Greater South Bay Health Plan [Torrance]	1,943		Network	1	P	NFQ
Health Net [Woodland Hills]	762,000		Network	10	NP	FQ
Inter Valley Health Plan [Pomona]	34,671		IPA	10	NP	FQ
Kaiser Fdn. Health Plan, Inc./So. CA Region [Pasadena]	2,236,511[a]	7,966	Group	44	NP	FQ
Maxicare California	121,000		IPA	17	P	FQ
MetLife HealthCare Network of So. CA, Inc.	64,822		IPA	3	P	NFQ
Ross-Loos Medical Group* [Glendale]	326,563	1,691	Staff	60	P	NFQ

STATE HMO Metro Location Plan Name [Headquarters City]	Pure Members	Open-ended Members	Model Type	Plan Age	Profit Status	Qual Status
CALIFORNIA *(Cont'd)*						
Los Angeles-Long Beach, CA *(Cont'd)*						
SCAN Health Plan	1,981		IPA	4	NP	NFQ
United Health Plan [Inglewood]	56,374		Network	16	NP	FQ
Universal Care	25,000		Staff	5	P	NFQ
Modesto, CA						
National Med	27,069		IPA	4	P	FQ
Oakland, CA						
CIGNA Health Plan of No. California, Inc.	3,684	1,813	IPA	2	P	NFQ
HEALS, The Personal Care Physician Hlth. Plan	95,500		IPA	8	P	FQ
Kaiser Fdn. Health Plan, Inc./No. CA Region	2,402,539[a]		Group	44	NP	FQ
TakeCare Corporation [Concord]	229,000		Network	11	P	FQ
Oxnard-Ventura, CA						
VIP Health Plan	29,392		IPA	7	P	FQ

Riverside-San Bernardino, CA

PARTNERS Health Plan of So. CA - Aetna	110,511		IPA	8	P	FQ

Sacramento, CA

Foundation Health [Rancho Cordova]	262,900		IPA	12	P	FQ
PCA Health Plans of California	16,695[b]		Group	14	P	FQ
Travelers Health Network of California, Inc.	3,613		IPA	4	P	FQ

San Diego, CA

CHOICE Healthcare Plan - Aetna	65,000		IPA	5	P	NFQ
CIGNA Healthplan of So. California, Inc.	33,801	661	IPA	6	P	FQ
Community Health Group [Chula Vista]	8,599		Network	3	NP	NFQ
Lincoln National Health Plan, Inc. (CA)* [Pleasonton]	94,790		Group	10	P	FQ

San Francisco, CA

Bay Pacific Health Plan [San Bruno]	115,074		IPA	10	P	FQ
Bridgeway Plan For Health	57,000		Network	14	P	FQ
Chinese Community Health Plan	5,064		IPA	2	P	NFQ
Contra Costa Health Plan [Martinez]	16,896		Staff	15	NP	FQ

As of 07/01/90

STATE HMO Metro Location Plan Name [Headquarters City]	Pure Members	Open-ended Members	Model Type	Plan Age	Profit Status	Qual Status
CALIFORNIA *(Cont'd)*						
San Francisco, CA *(Cont'd)*						
Golden Bay Health Plan	383		Network	1	P	NFQ
The Blue Shield HMO	10,444		Network	1	NP	NFQ
San Jose, CA						
Coast Health Plan [Los Altos]	2,005		IPA	1	NP	NFQ
Health Plan Plus [Alviso]	11,950		Staff	15	NP	NFQ
Lifeguard HMO	140,000[b]		IPA	10	NP	FQ
Valley Health Plan	2,998		Staff	4	NP	NFQ
Santa Barbara-Santa Maria-Lompoc, CA						
Freedom Plan, Inc.	7,800		IPA	2	P	NFQ
Santa Rosa-Petaluma, CA						
Health Plan of the Redwoods	70,000		IPA	9	NP	FQ
Stockton, CA						
St. Joseph's OMNI Health Plan	25,000		IPA	3	P	FQ

COLORADO

Colorado Springs, CO

Plan			Model	#		
Health Network of Colorado Springs	9,359		IPA	3	P	FQ
Lincoln Health Plan of Colorado, LTD* [Denver]	103,345		Network	10	P	FQ
Qual-Med Colorado Springs HMO	6,247	1,055	IPA	3	P	FQ

Denver, CO

Plan			Model	#		
CIGNA Healthplan of Colorado, Inc.	4,502	1,034	IPA	3	P	FQ
Comprecare Colorado [Aurora]	157,438	11,255	IPA	15	P	FQ
Exclusive Health Care of Colorado, Inc. [Omaha]	1,072		Network	<1	P	NFQ
HMO Colorado	60,782		Network	10	P	FQ
Humana Health Plan, Inc.	2,409[a]		IPA	<1	P	NFQ
Kaiser Fdn. Health Plan of Colorado	238,878[a]		Group	20	NP	FQ
MetLife HealthCare Network of Colorado, Inc.	15,427		IPA	3	P	NFQ
PARTNERS Health Plan of Colorado - Aetna [Englewood]	7,336		IPA	2	P	NFQ
PruCare of Colorado	244[b]		IPA	3	P	FQ

STATE HMO Metro Location Plan Name [Headquarters City]	Pure Members	Open-ended Members	Model Type	Plan Age	Profit Status	Qual Status
COLORADO *(Cont'd)*						
Denver, CO *(Cont'd)*						
Qual-Med Greater Denver HMO [Aurora]	1,244	731	IPA	3	P	FQ
Pueblo, CO						
Qual-Med Pueblo HMO	4,784		IPA	6	P	FQ
Qual-Med Upper Arkansas Valley HMO	518	11	IPA	3	P	FQ
Southern Colorado Health Plan	6,710		IPA	3	P	NFQ
Non-Metropolitan						
Rocky Mountain HMO [Grand Junction]	38,110		IPA	16	NP	FQ
San Luis Valley HMO [Monte Vista]	6,258		IPA	14	NP	FQ
CONNECTICUT						
Bridgeport-Milford, CT						
Physicians Health Services of CT, Inc. [Trumbull]	127,126		IPA	12	P	FQ

Plan	Enrollment		Model	No.		
Suburban Health Plan [Shelton]	1,950		IPA	1	P	NFQ
U.S. Healthcare [Shelton]	12,500[a]		IPA	2	P	FQ
Hartford, CT						
CIGNA Healthplan of Connecticut [East Hartford]	34,779	11,183	IPA	3	P	FQ
ConnectiCare [Farmington]	95,889		IPA	7	NP	FQ
Kaiser Perm. Medical Care Program/NE Region [Farmington]	112,349[a]		Group	13	NP	FQ
PARTNERS Hlth Pl of So. New England - Aetna [Hamden]	19,051		IPA	2	NP	NFQ
New Haven-Meriden, CT						
Community Health Care Plan, Inc.	53,615		Staff	18	NP	FQ
Constitution HealthCare, Inc.* [North Haven]	115,524		IPA	11	NP	FQ
M.D. Health Plan [North Haven]	42,648	87	IPA	2	P	NFQ
Yale Health Plan	25,307[a]		Staff	18	NP	NFQ
Norwalk, CT						
PruCare of Connecticut	2,621		IPA	1	P	FQ

As of 07/01/90

STATE HMO Metro Location Plan Name [Headquarters City]	Pure Members	Open-ended Members	Model Type	Plan Age	Profit Status	Qual Status
DELAWARE						
Wilmington, DE-NJ-MD						
CIGNA Healthplan of Delaware [Lester]	10,170	1,570	IPA	4	P	FQ
Healthcare Delaware, Inc.	22,603		IPA	3	P	NFQ
Principal HealthCare of Delaware, Inc. [Newark]	27,000	2,200	IPA	3	P	NFQ
The HMO of Delaware [Newark]	19,369		Staff	6	P	NFQ
Total Health, Inc. [Newark]	30,806		IPA	4	P	NFQ
U.S. Healthcare	7,500[a]		IPA	2	P	FQ
DISTRICT OF COLUMBIA						
Washington, DC-MD-VA						
George Washington University Health Plan	45,697		Network	17	NP	FQ
Group Health Association	154,551		Staff	52	NP	FQ

Kaiser Fdn. Hlth Pl, Inc./Mid-Atlantic Region	284,495[a]		Group	17	NP	FQ
PruCare of Washington D.C. [Bethesda]	1,296		IPA	<1	P	NFQ

FLORIDA

Daytona Beach, FL

Florida Health Care Plan, Inc.	23,706		Staff	15	P	FQ

Ft. Lauderdale-Hollywood-Pompano Beach, FL

CIGNA Healthplan of South Florida [Miami Lakes]	10,585	2,818	IPA	15	P	FQ
HIP Network of Florida	19,172		IPA	4	NP	NFQ
PruCare of South Florida	6,850		IPA	3	P	FQ

Jacksonville, FL

Anthem Health Plans of Florida, Inc.*	8,668		IPA	2	P	NFQ
Health Options	207,000	4,700	IPA	9	P	FQ
Principal Health Care of Florida, Inc.	19,700		IPA	5	P	NFQ
PruCare of Jacksonville	36,366		Group	5	P	FQ

Lakeland-Winter Haven, FL

Florida 1st Health Plan	12,543		IPA	3	P	NFQ

STATE HMO Metro Location Plan Name [Headquarters City]	Pure Members	Open-ended Members	Model Type	Plan Age	Profit Status	Qual Status
FLORIDA *(Cont'd)*						
Miami-Hialeah, FL						
Association I.N.E.D.	7,680[d]		Staff	4	P	NFQ
Av-Med Health Plan	170,808	39,281	IPA	12	NP	FQ
CAC-Ramsay, Inc. [Coral Gables]	66,118		Staff	19	P	FQ
Century Medical Center, Inc.	61,488[c]		IPA	3	P	NFQ
Family Health Plan, Inc. [Miami Lakes]	31,235		IPA	2	P	NFQ
Heritage Health Plan of South Florida	22,610		IPA	4	P	NFQ
Humana Medical Plan, Inc.	373,899[o]		Network	17	P	FQ
JMH Health Plan	8,569		Staff	4	NP	NFQ
Pasteur Health Plan HMO, Inc.	20,210		Staff	4	P	NFQ
Patient Care of America	1,819		IPA	2	P	NFQ
Preferred Medical Health Plan*	10,200		Staff	17	P	NFQ

Orlando, FL

Name			Model		P/NP	FQ
CIGNA Healthplan of Florida, Inc. [Maitland]	12,283	6,880	Mixed^r	6	P	FQ
MetLife HealthCare Network of Florida, Inc. [Maitland]	28,088		IPA	3	P	FQ
PruCare of Orlando [Maitland]	44,091		Group	6	P	FQ

Pensacola, FL

Name			Model		P/NP	FQ
Medical Center Health Plan	10,207		Network	4	P	NFQ

Tallahassee, FL

Name			Model		P/NP	FQ
Capital Health Plan	42,700		Staff	7	NP	FQ
Healthplan Southeast	27,006		IPA	3	P	NFQ

Tampa-St. Petersburg-Clearwater, FL

Name			Model		P/NP	FQ
CIGNA Healthplan of Florida, Inc.	27,475	4,071	Mixed^r	11	P	FQ
PARTNERS Health Plan of FL - Aetna	12,402		IPA	1	P	NFQ
PruCare of Tampa Bay	14,628		IPA	4	P	FQ

GEORGIA

Atlanta, GA

Name			Model		P/NP	FQ
CIGNA Healthplan of Georgia	32,702	3,139	IPA	8	P	FQ
Health 1st	51,800	16,400	IPA	10	P	FQ

As of 07/01/90

STATE HMO Metro Location Plan Name [Headquarters City]	Pure Members	Open-ended Members	Model Type	Plan Age	Profit Status	Qual Status
GEORGIA *(Cont'd)*						
Atlanta, GA *(Cont'd)*						
HMO Georgia, Inc.	8,000[f]		IPA	3	P	NFQ
Kaiser Fdn. Health Plan of Georgia, Inc.	136,070[a]		Group	4	NP	FQ
MetLife HealthCare Network of Georgia, Inc.	2,629		IPA	2	P	NFQ
PARTNERS Health Plan of Georgia - Aetna	32,786		Network	3	P	FQ
PruCare of Atlanta	39,438		Group	8	P	FQ
Augusta, GA-SC						
Master Health Plan	4,954		Mixed[t]	2	P	NFQ
GUAM						
Non-Metropolitan						
FHP, Inc. [Tamuning]	29,737[l]		Staff	16	P	FQ
Guam Memorial Health Plan [Agana]	26,000[b]		IPA	12	NP	NFQ

Health Maintenance Life Insurance Co. [Tamuning]	4,077	IPA	15	P	NFQ

HAWAII

Honolulu, HI

Community Health Program	18,709	Network	17	NP	NFQ
Health Plan Hawaii	18,288	Network	8	NP	FQ
Island Care	22,919	Group^u	9	NP	NFQ
Kaiser Fdn. Health Plan, Inc./Hawaii Region	177,924[a]	Group	31	NP	FQ
Pacific Health Care	2,637	IPA	1	NP	NFQ

IDAHO

Boise City, ID

Lincoln National Health Plan, Inc.	17,804	Group	4	P	FQ

ILLINOIS

Aurora-Elgin, IL

Dreyer HMO	28,763	Group	5	NP	FQ

Champaign-Urbana-Rantoul, IL

CarleCare	62,306	Network	10	P	FQ
PersonalCare HMO	37,541	Network	5	P	FQ

As of 07/01/90

STATE HMO Metro Location Plan Name [Headquarters City]	Pure Members	Open-ended Members	Model Type	Plan Age	Profit Status	Qual Status
ILLINOIS *(Cont'd)*						
Chicago, IL						
American HMO [Flossmoor]	23,142		Network	5	P	NFQ
Chicago HMO Ltd.	175,890		Network	13	P	FQ
CIGNA Healthplan of Illinois, Inc. [Des Plaines]	18,907	2,387	IPA	3	P	FQ
COMPASS Health Care Plans	16,688		Network[v]	5	NP	NFQ
Great Lakes Health Plan, Inc. [Lombard]	47,437[e]		IPA	4	P	FQ
HealthChicago, Inc. [Lisle]	61,565		IPA	5	P	FQ
HMO Illinois	307,584		Network	12	NP	FQ
Illinois Masonic Community Health Plan	2,823		Network	4	NP	NFQ
Maxicare Illinois, Inc.	31,000		IPA	17	P	FQ
Med Care [Maywood]	38,477		IPA	4	NP	NFQ

Plan	Enrollment		Model	Physicians		
MetLife HealthCare Network of Illinois, Inc. [Schaumburg]	19,727		IPA	3	P	NFQ
Michael Reese Health Plan	237,475		Staff	17	NP	FQ
MultiCare HMO	6,600		Network	5	P	NFQ
PARTNERS Health Plan of Illinois - Aetna*	14,858		IPA	7	P	NFQ
PruCare of Illinois [Rosemont]	27,627		Group	15	P	FQ
Rush Access	44,522		IPA	3	P	NFQ
Rush-Presbyterian St. Luke's Health Plans	126,098		Staff	18	NP	FQ
SHARE Health Plan of Illinois [Itasca]	55,000	230	Network	5	P	FQ
Union Health Service	27,019[c]		Staff	34	NP	NFQ
University of Illinois HMO	4,500		Group	3	NP	NFQ
Joliet, IL						
Complete Health Care Corporation	2,531[b]		IPA	4	P	NFQ
Peoria, IL						
Health Plan of Central Illinois	26,875		IPA	6	P	NFQ
Rockford, IL						
CliniCare [Loves Park]	24,883		Network	9	P	FQ

As of 07/01/90

STATE HMO Metro Location Plan Name [Headquarters City]	Pure Members	Open-ended Members	Model Type	Plan Age	Profit Status	Qual Status
INDIANA						
Evansville, IN-KY						
Physicians Health Network, Inc.	19,278		IPA	4	P	FQ
Welborn HMO, A Division of Welborn Clinic	33,143		Group	3	P	FQ
Fort Wayne, IN						
Physicians Health Plan of No. Indiana	43,300		IPA	6	NP	FQ
Gary-Hammond, IN						
HMO America-Indiana, Inc. [Chicago]	1,811		Network	4	P	NFQ
Indianapolis, IN						
Farm Bureau Insurance Health Care Network	15,278		IPA	3	P	NFQ
Health Maintenance of Indiana	42,239		IPA	6	P	FQ
Lincoln National Health Plan, Inc. [Fort Wayne]	40,235		IPA	4	P	FQ
M Plan	11,174		IPA	<1	P	NFQ
Maxicare Indiana	82,000		IPA	11	P	FQ

Lafayette, IN

Arnett HMO	19,220		Group	4	P	FQ

South Bend-Mishawaka, IN

PARTNERS Health Plan - Aetna	29,848		IPA	3	P	NFQ

Non-Metropolitan

Southeastern Indiana Health Organization [Columbus]	1,500		IPA	2	NP	NFQ

IOWA

Davenport-Rock Island-Moline, IA-IL

Heritage National Healthplan, Inc.	169,501		IPA	3	P	NFQ

Des Moines, IA

Family Health Plan	5,258		IPA	4	P	NFQ
HMO Iowa	28,428		IPA	4	P	NFQ
SHARE Health Plan of Iowa [West Des Moines]	26,154	87	Network	6	P	FQ
Total Health Network of Iowa, Inc.	23,390		Network	5	P	NFQ

Dubuque, IA

Medical Associates Health Plan, Inc.	27,080		Group	7	P	FQ

As of 07/01/90

STATE HMO Metro Location Plan Name [Headquarters City]	Pure Members	Open-ended Members	Model Type	Plan Age	Profit Status	Qual Status
IOWA (Cont'd)						
Sioux City, IA-NE						
Care Choices of Iowa	6,467		IPA	2	NP	NFQ
KANSAS						
Kansas City, MO-KS						
CIGNA Healthplan of Kansas City, Inc. [Overland Park]	15,982	612	IPA	3	P	FQ
Kaiser Fdn. Health Plan of Kansas City [Shawnee Mission]	43,220[a]		Group	7	NP	FQ
MetLife HlthCare Network of Kansas City, Inc. [Overland Park]	2,692		IPA	2	P	NFQ
Preferred Medical/Medplan [Overland Park]	15,239		Network[x]	4	P	NFQ
Topeka, KS						
HMO Kansas	49,926		IPA	5	NP	NFQ

Wichita, KS

	Enrollment		Model			
EQUICOR Health Plan, Inc.	60,259		IPA	8	P	FQ

Non-Metropolitan

EQUICOR [Salina]	4,957		IPA	6	P	FQ
Family Health Plan Corporation [Newton]	7,076		Network	8	P	FQ

KENTUCKY

Lexington-Fayette, KY

HealthWise of Kentucky, Ltd.	34,454		IPA	3	P	NFQ
Humana Care Plan, Inc.	37,558[a]		IPA	16	P	FQ

Louisville, KY-IN

Alternative Health Delivery System*	30,000		IPA	3	P	NFQ
HMO Kentucky	44,727[c]		IPA	4	P	FQ
Humana Health Plan, Inc.	56,528[p]	88,123	IPA	4	P	FQ
MetLife HealthCare Network of Kentucky, Inc.	68		IPA	4	P	NFQ

Non-Metropolitan

Choice Care of Kentucky, Inc. [Crestview Hills]	7,654		IPA	3	NP	NFQ

As of 07/01/90

STATE HMO Metro Location Plan Name [Headquarters City]	Pure Members	Open-ended Members	Model Type	Plan Age	Profit Status	Qual Status
LOUISIANA						
Baton Rouge, LA						
CIGNA Healthplan of Louisiana, Inc.	12,032	3,800	IPA	3	P	FQ
Community Health Network of Louisiana, Inc.	35,267		IPA	2	P	FQ
Gulf South Health Plans, Inc.	20,071		IPA	3	P	NFQ
New Orleans, LA						
Maxicare Louisiana, Inc. [Metairie]	19,000		Network[V]	5	P	FQ
Ochsner Health Plan [Metairie]	83,833		Group	4	P	FQ
PARTNERS Health Plan of Louisiana - Aetna [Metairie]	6,017		IPA	2	P	NFQ
Principal Health Care of Louisiana, Inc. [Metairie]	30,500	700	IPA	4	P	FQ
Travelers Health Network of Louisiana, Inc. [Metairie]	14,485		IPA	4	P	FQ

Shreveport, LA

Plan			Model			
CIGNA Healthplan of Northern Louisiana	16,141	1,623	Mixed[t]	5	P	FQ

MAINE

Portland, ME

Plan			Model			
Healthsource Maine, Inc. [Yarmouth]	9,000		IPA	2	P	FQ
HMO Maine	12,594[g]		IPA	18	NP	FQ
Lincoln National Health Plan, Inc. [S. Portland]	10,454		IPA	2	P	NFQ

MARYLAND

Baltimore, MD

Plan			Model			
Chesapeake Health Plan	21,015		Network	12	NP	NFQ
CIGNA Healthplan of Mid-Atlantic, Inc. [Columbia]	11,965	5,320	IPA	3	P	FQ
HealthCare Corporation of the Mid-Atlantic*	6,755[c]		Network	12	P	FQ
HealthCare Corporation of the Potomac*	13,792[c]		Network	5	P	NFQ
The Columbia Free State Health System [Columbia]	185,700		Network	20	P	FQ
The Johns Hopkins Health Plan	92,114	2,318	IPA	5	NP	FQ
Total HealthCare	22,683		Staff	17	NP	FQ

STATE HMO Metro Location Plan Name [Headquarters City]	Pure Members	Open-ended Members	Model Type	Plan Age	Profit Status	Qual Status
MARYLAND *(Cont'd)*						
Washington, DC–MD–VA						
HealthPlus [Riverdale]	119,726	22,131	IPA	11	P	FQ
Lincoln National Health Plan, Inc. [Bethesda]	8,078[c]		IPA	3	P	NFQ
M.D. IPA Health Plan [Rockville]	164,000	35,000	IPA	9	P	FQ
Non-Metropolitan						
Delmarva Health Care Plan [Easton]	21,000		IPA	7	P	NFQ
MASSACHUSETTS						
Boston, MA						
Bay State Health Care [Cambridge]	315,730		IPA	10	NP	FQ
Harvard Community Health Plan [Brookline]	415,336		Staff	20	NP	FQ

Plan						
Harvard Univ. Group Health Program [Cambridge]	5,970		Staff	17	NP	NFQ
Lahey Clinic - BC/BS HMP [Cambridge]	24,132		Group	9	NP	NFQ
Medical West Community Health Plan [Framingham]	147,433		Staff	11	NP	FQ
MetLife HealthCare Network of MA, Inc. [Canton]	1,678		IPA	2	P	NFQ
MIT Health Plans [Cambridge]	8,103	1,523	Staff	16	NP	NFQ
Neighborhood Health Plan [Dorchester]	15,000		Network	2	NP	NFQ
Pilgrim Health Care [Norwell]	149,905		IPA	8	NP	FQ
Tufts Associated Health Plan [Waltham]	121,579		IPA	8	NP	FQ
U.S. Healthcare [Waltham]	20,000[a]		IPA	2	P	NFQ
Fitchburg-Leominster, MA						
Montachusett Health Plan	8,171		IPA	5	NP	NFQ
Pittsfield, MA						
Berkshire Health Plan	32,449		IPA	5	NP	NFQ

STATE HMO Metro Location Plan Name [Headquarters City]	Pure Members	Open-ended Members	Model Type	Plan Age	Profit Status	Qual Status
MASSACHUSETTS *(Cont'd)*						
Salem-Gloucester, MA						
North Shore Health Plan [Cambridge]	10,575		IPA	4	NP	NFQ
Springfield, MA						
CIGNA Healthplan of Massachusetts, Inc.	15,955	790	IPA	3	P	FQ
Health New England	33,000		IPA	4	P	FQ
Worcester, MA						
Central Massachusetts Health Care	100,030		IPA	10	NP	NFQ
Fallon Community Health Plan [West Boylston]	125,969		Group	12	NP	FQ
Non-Metropolitan						
Community Health Plan of Massachusetts - CHP [West Springfield]	16,036ʲ		Network	6	NP	FQ

MICHIGAN

Ann Arbor, MI

Plan	Enrollment		Model		NP/P	FQ/NFQ
Care Choices Health Plans [Farmington Hills]	102,869		IPA	5	NP	NFQ
M-Care	35,700		Network	3	NP	NFQ

Detroit, MI

Plan	Enrollment		Model		NP/P	FQ/NFQ
Blue Care Network of Southeast Michigan [Southfield]	99,790		IPA	8	NP	FQ
Comprehensive Health Services of Detroit	74,816		Staff	16	NP	FQ
Health Alliance Plan of Michigan	386,888	11,047	Group	29	NP	FQ
OmniCare Health Plan	84,904		Network	15	NP	FQ
SelectCare MedExtend [Troy]	80,740	1,693	Staff	12	P	FQ
Total Health Care, Inc.	18,212		IPA	16	NP	FQ

Flint, MI

Plan	Enrollment		Model		NP/P	FQ/NFQ
HealthPlus of Michigan	89,941		IPA	10	NP	FQ

Grand Rapids, MI

Plan	Enrollment		Model		NP/P	FQ/NFQ
Blue Care Network, Great Lakes	107,884		Network	7	NP	FQ
Butterworth HMO, a PRTNRS Hlth Pl - Aetna	45,357		IPA	3	NP	NFQ
Grand Valley Health Plan	19,100		Staff	7	P	NFQ

Lansing-East Lansing, MI

Plan	Enrollment		Model		NP/P	FQ/NFQ
Blue Care Network - Health Central	66,706		Network	12	NP	FQ

As of 07/01/90

STATE HMO Metro Location Plan Name [Headquarters City]	Pure Members	Open-ended Members	Model Type	Plan Age	Profit Status	Qual Status
MICHIGAN *(Cont'd)*						
Lansing-East Lansing, MI *(Cont'd)*						
Physicians Health Plan	106,153	14,546	IPA	8	NP	FQ
Saginaw-Bay City-Midland, MI						
Blue Care Network of East Michigan	66,633		Network	14	NP	FQ
Non-Metropolitan						
LakeShore HMO [Holland]	17,780		IPA	4	P	NFQ
North Med HMO [Traverse City]	4,525		IPA	2	P	NFQ
MINNESOTA						
Minneapolis/St. Paul, MN-WI						
Blue Plus	24,205	52,847	IPA	15	NP	FQ
Group Health, Inc.	214,214	63,701	Staff	32	NP	FQ
MedCenters Health Plan - Aetna [St. Louis Park]	229,042	33,100	Network	17	NP	NFQ

Metropolitan Health Plan	15,000	5,000	Group	5	NP	NFQ
NWNL Health Network	5,600	12,447	Network	5	NP	NFQ
Physicians Health Plan of Minnesota	54,678	211,158	IPA	14	NP	NFQ
SHARE Health Plan [Bloomington]	141,387		Network	15	NP	NFQ
UCare Minnesota	1,848		Network	<1	NP	NFQ
Rochester, MN						
Mayo Health Plan	4,461		Network	3	NP	NFQ
St. Cloud, MN						
Central Minnesota Group Health Plan	16,226	678	Staff	10	NP	FQ
Non-Metropolitan						
First Plan HMO/Community Health Center [Two Harbors]	5,712	2,710	Mixed[s]	45	NP	NFQ
MISSOURI						
Kansas City, MO-KS						
Blue Care	5,305		IPA	1	NP	NFQ
Lincoln National Hlth Pl of Kansas City,Inc.	2,713		IPA	2	P	NFQ
Prime Health	80,773		Staff	13	P	FQ
Principal Health Care of Kansas City, Inc.	22,000	1,500	IPA	1	P	NFQ

STATE HMO Metro Location Plan Name [Headquarters City]	Pure Members	Open-ended Members	Model Type	Plan Age	Profit Status	Qual Status
MISSOURI *(Cont'd)*						
Kansas City, MO-KS *(Cont'd)*						
PruCare of Kansas City	3,068		IPA	3	P	NFQ
Total Health Care	46,932		IPA	8	NP	FQ
St. Louis, MO-IL						
BlueChoice	55,000		IPA	2	P	FQ
CIGNA Healthplan of St. Louis [Clayton]	10,401	2,560	IPA	4	P	FQ
HealthAmerica*	117,750		Staff	8	P	FQ
Lincoln National Health Plan, Inc.	1,935		IPA	2	P	NFQ
MetLife HealthCare Network, Inc. [St.Louis]	33,819		IPA	21	P	NFQ
PARTNERS HMO - Aetna	19,298		IPA	1	NP	NFQ
Physicians Health Plan of Greater St. Louis	13,098	14,137	IPA	3	P	FQ
PruCare of St. Louis [Creve Coeur]	14,529		IPA	4	P	FQ

Sanus Health Plan	96,249	IPA	4	P	FQ
St. Louis Labor Health Institute	11,280	Staff	44	NP	NFQ

Non-Metropolitan

CarePlus of Missouri, Inc. [Rolla]	7,600	IPA	3	P	NFQ

MONTANA

Non-Metropolitan

HMO Montana [Helena]	5,200	IPA	2	NP	NFQ

NEBRASKA

Lincoln, NE

HealthAmerica/CapitalCare, Inc.	14,300	Staff	10	NP	FQ

Omaha, NE-IA

Exclusive Health Care, Inc.	11,064	IPA	1	P	NFQ
HMO Nebraska	17,902	IPA	4	P	FQ
Principal Health Care of Nebraska, Inc.	10,000	IPA	3	P	NFQ
SHARE Health Plan of Nebraska	29,000	IPA	5	P	FQ

As of 07/01/90

STATE HMO Metro Location Plan Name [Headquarters City]	Pure Members	Open-ended Members	Model Type	Plan Age	Profit Status	Qual Status
NEVADA						
Las Vegas, NV						
Health Plan of Nevada - Las Vegas	65,651	6,719	Group	6	P	FQ
Humana Medical Plan of Nevada, Inc.	1,104[a]		IPA	<1	P	NFQ
Reno, NV						
Hospital Health Plan	27,800		IPA	1	NP	FQ
NEW HAMPSHIRE						
Nashua, NH						
Matthew Thornton Health Plan	66,450		Network	18	NP	FQ
Non-Metropolitan						
Healthsource New Hampshire [Concord]	39,792	500	IPA	4	P	FQ
NEW JERSEY						
Atlantic City, NJ						
PruCare of New Jersey [Parsippany]	72,169		IPA	12	P	FQ

Bergen-Passaic, NJ						
CIGNA Healthplan of No. New Jersey [Paramus]	2,735	2,682	IPA	1	P	NFQ
HMO of New Jersey, Inc. [Paramus]	378,000[a]		IPA	6	P	FQ
Middlesex-Somerset-Hunterdon, NJ						
Aetna Health Plans of New Jersey* [Iselin]	136,916		IPA	8	P	FQ
Rutgers Community Health Plan	86,602	167	Group	13	P	FQ
Monmouth-Ocean, NJ						
Medigroup - Shoreline [Cranford]	15,869		IPA	4	P	NFQ
New York, NY						
Oxford Health Plans of New Jersey	2,436	3,980	IPA	4	P	FQ
Newark, NJ						
Medigroup - Metro [Cranford]	12,929		IPA	3	P	NFQ
Medigroup - North [Cranford]	2,582		IPA	3	P	NFQ
Total Health of New Jersey [New York]	88,097		IPA	11	P	FQ

STATE HMO Metro Location Plan Name [Headquarters City]	Pure Members	Open-ended Members	Model Type	Plan Age	Profit Status	Qual Status
NEW JERSEY *(Cont'd)*						
Philadelphia, PA-NJ						
CIGNA Healthplan of Southern New Jersey [Lester]	13,997	4,732	IPA	4	P	FQ
HIP of New Jersey [Somerset]	81,988	735	Group	13	NP	FQ
Medigroup - South [Cranford]	14,934		IPA	3	P	NFQ
Trenton, NJ						
Medigroup - Central, Inc.	26,939		Mixed[r]	16	P	NFQ
Vineland-Millville-Bridgeton, NJ						
OMNICARE/the HMO, Inc.	18,882		Network	14	P	NFQ
NEW MEXICO						
Albuquerque, NM						
EQUICOR, Inc.	109,000		Group	17	P	FQ
FHP of New Mexico, Inc.	27,193		IPA	3	P	FQ

	FIRSTSOURCE					
FIRSTSOURCE	12,500		IPA	4	P	FQ
Health Plus of New Mexico	28,095		IPA	3	P	FQ
Qual-Med New Mexico Health Plan	17,877	393	IPA	5	P	FQ
NEW YORK						
Albany-Schenectady-Troy, NY						
Capital District Physicians Health Plan	94,744		IPA	5	NP	NFQ
Community Health Plan - CHP [Latham]	73,506		Staff	13	NP	FQ
Mohawk Valley Physicians Health Plan - East	60,327		IPA	6	NP	NFQ
Buffalo, NY						
Community Blue, The HMO of BC of Western NY	126,956		IPA	4	NP	NFQ
Health Care Plan	72,916	2,052	Staff	11	NP	FQ
Independent Health	140,783		IPA	9	NP	FQ
Nassau-Suffolk, NY						
ChoiceCare - Long Island [Uniondale]	22,926		IPA	4	NP	NFQ
MetLife HealthCare Network of New York, Inc. [Lake Success]	20,212		IPA	2	P	NFQ
Total Health of New York [New York]	35,863		IPA	3	P	FQ

As of 07/01/90

STATE HMO Metro Location Plan Name [Headquarters City]	Pure Members	Open-ended Members	Model Type	Plan Age	Profit Status	Qual Status
NEW YORK *(Cont'd)*						
Nassau-Suffolk, NY *(Cont'd)*						
U.S. Healthcare [Lake Success]	120,000^a		IPA	3	P	FQ
New York, NY						
Aetna Health Plans of New York - Aetna* [Tarrytown]	9,213		IPA	3	P	NFQ
Elderplan, Inc. [Brooklyn]	5,119		Group^y	4	NP	NFQ
Empire Blue Cross & Blue Shield HEALTHNET	186,784		IPA^t	17	NP	NFQ
Health Insurance Plan of Greater New York	879,445	21,666	Group	42	NP	NFQ
Independent Health [Tarrytown]	11,582		IPA	3	NP	FQ
Metropolitan Health Plan	3,686^c		Group	4	NP	NFQ
Oxford Health Plans of New York	19,498	20,416	IPA	3	P	NFQ
Physicians Health Services of New York [Hartsdale]	8,353		IPA	2	P	FQ

Plan						
PruCare of New York [Hauppauge]	34,835		IPA	2	P	NFQ
Sanus Health Plan of New York & New Jersey	27,917	20,108	IPA	3	P	FQ
Travelers Health Network of New York, Inc. [White Plains]	7,962		IPA	3	P	FQ
WellCare of New York, Inc. [Newburgh]	16,500		IPA	2	P	NFQ
Poughkeepsie, NY						
HealthShield - CHP	34,000[j]		Staff	7	NP	FQ
Mohawk Valley Phys. Health Plan - Mid Hudson	11,599		IPA	1	NP	FQ
Rochester, NY						
Blue Choice	284,751		IPA	5	NP	NFQ
Genesee Valley Group Health	50,852[h]		Group	16	NP	NFQ
Preferred Care	153,000		IPA	10	NP	FQ
Syracuse, NY						
Health Svcs. Med. Corp of Central New York [Baldwinsville]	51,730		Group	12	NP	FQ
HMO-CNY, Inc. [Baldwinsville]	40,294		IPA	5	P	NFQ
Patients' Choice, Inc.	26,619		IPA	3	P	NFQ
Travelers Health Network of New York, Inc.	18,093		IPA	4	P	FQ

As of 07/01/90

STATE HMO Metro Location Plan Name [Headquarters City]	Pure Members	Open-ended Members	Model Type	Plan Age	Profit Status	Qual Status
NEW YORK *(Cont'd)*						
Utica-Rome, NY						
BlueCARE Plus	13,500		IPA	3	NP	NFQ
Mohawk Valley Physicians Health Plan-Central [Yorkville]	14,257		IPA	3	NP	NFQ
Non-Metropolitan						
Community Health Plan of Bassett - CHP [Cooperstown]	7,589		Network[x]	3	NP	NFQ
Mid-Hudson Health Plan [Kingston]	16,600		IPA	5	NP	NFQ
Mohawk Valley Phys Health Plan - So. Central [Schenectady]	2,137		IPA	1	NP	NFQ
Mohawk Valley Physicians Health Plan - North [Schenectady]	5,777		IPA	1	NP	NFQ
NORTH CAROLINA						
Charlotte-Gastonia-Rock Hill, NC-SC						
PruCare of Charlotte	33,901		Group	4	P	FQ

Greensboro-Winston-Salem-High Point, NC

PARTNERS National Health Plans of NC - Aetna	29,247	5,000	IPA	3	P	NFQ
Physicians Health Plan of North Carolina	30,600		IPA	4	P	NFQ
Winston-Salem Health Care Plan	35,022		Staff	13	NP	NFQ

Raleigh-Durham, NC

Blue Cross & Blue Shield/Personal Care Plan	11,712		IPA	7	NP	NFQ
Carolina Physicians' Health Plan, Inc.	36,937		IPA	3	P	NFQ
EQUICOR, Inc.	1,113		IPA	3	P	NFQ
HMO of North Carolina, Inc.	9,325		Group	3	P	NFQ
Kaiser Fdn. Health Plan of North Carolina	103,398[a]		Group	5	NP	FQ
Lincoln National Health Plan, Inc.	1,982		IPA	1	P	NFQ
Maxicare North Carolina, Inc. [Charlotte]	10,000		IPA	5	P	FQ
Personal Care Plan of North Carolina, Inc.	11,874		IPA	4	P	FQ

NORTH DAKOTA

Fargo-Moorhead, ND-MN

Care Plan HMO	7,860[b]		IPA	4	NP	FQ

As of 07/01/90

STATE HMO Metro Location Plan Name [Headquarters City]	Pure Members	Open-ended Members	Model Type	Plan Age	Profit Status	Qual Status
NORTH DAKOTA *(Cont'd)*						
Non-Metropolitan						
Heart of America HMO [Rugby]	3,150		Group	7	NP	FQ
OHIO						
Cincinnati, OH-KY-IN						
ChoiceCare	133,794		IPA	10	NP	FQ
Community Health Plan of Ohio - CHP	12,702		Network^w	3	NP	NFQ
Health Maintenance Plan	119,844		Network	15	NP	NFQ
Lincoln National Health Plan, Inc.	30,944		Network	5	P	FQ
Magna Care Health Plan	20,988		IPA	3	NP	NFQ
PruCare of Cincinnati	4,774		IPA	3	P	NFQ
University Health Plan	25,882		IPA	3	NP	NFQ
Cleveland, OH						
CIGNA Healthplan of Ohio	14,888	1,644	IPA	2	P	FQ

Plan	Enrollment		Model	No.		
HMO Health Ohio	116,290		Network	11	P	NFQ
Kaiser Fdn. Health Plan of Ohio	207,025[a]		Group	25	NP	FQ
MetLife HealthCare Network of Ohio, Inc. [Cincinnati]	10,658		IPA	4	P	NFQ
PARTNERS Health Plan of No. Ohio - Aetna	44,717		IPA	6	P	NFQ
Personal Physician Care of Ohio, Inc.	17,943		IPA	2	NP	NFQ
PruCare of Cleveland	1,600		IPA	<1	P	NFQ
Total Health Care Plan	13,482		Group	2	NP	NFQ

Columbus, OH

Plan	Enrollment		Model	No.		
CIGNA Healthplan of Ohio	23,454	1,860	IPA	3	P	FQ
Health Power of Columbus*	29,000		Network	5	P	NFQ
Hospital Choice Health Plan [Worthington]	17,129		IPA	4	P	NFQ
Licking Memorial Hospital Health Plan [Newark]	14,511		IPA	3	NP	NFQ
Physicians Health Plan of Ohio	154,099		IPA	10	P	NFQ
Principal Health Care of Ohio, Inc.*	27,000		Group	8	P	NFQ
PruCare of Central Ohio	26,807		Group	4	P	FQ
United Health Plan	10,248		IPA	11	P	NFQ

STATE HMO Metro Location Plan Name [Headquarters City]	Pure Members	Open-ended Members	Model Type	Plan Age	Profit Status	Qual Status
OHIO *(Cont'd)*						
Dayton-Springfield, OH						
Day-Med Health Maintenance Plan	21,000		IPA	3	P	NFQ
Health Power	30,500		Network	4	P	NFQ
Western Ohio Health Care Plan	141,419q	4,056	IPA	11	P	NFQ
Toledo, OH						
Family Health Plan	19,000		IPA	4	NP	NFQ
MedChoice	54,194		IPA	5	P	NFQ
Medical Value Plan	41,560		IPA	3	P	NFQ
Paramount Care, Inc.	17,459		IPA	1	P	NFQ
The Toledo Health Plan	7,319		IPA	3	NP	NFQ
Wheeling, WV-OH						
HealthGuard [Bellaire]	7,389c		Group	15	NP	FQ

Non-Metropolitan

HealthOhio, Inc. [Marion]		28,683	IPA	13	NP	FQ
Hometown Hospital Health Plan [Massillon]		7,718	IPA	2	NP	NFQ

OKLAHOMA

Oklahoma City, OK

EQUICOR, Inc.		12,877	IPA	5	P	FQ
PacifiCare		34,321	Group	4	P	FQ
PruCare of Oklahoma City		22,323	Group	8	P	FQ

Tulsa, OK

BlueLincs HMO		38,755	IPA	5	P	FQ
PacifiCare of Oklahoma		47,808	Group	4	P	FQ
PruCare of Tulsa		20,075	Group	7	P	FQ

OREGON

Eugene-Springfield, OR

SelectCare	2,161	42,636[b]	IPA	10	NP	FQ

Medford, OR

Health Masters		6,145	IPA	2	P	FQ

As of 07/01/90

STATE HMO Metro Location Plan Name [Headquarters City]	Pure Members	Open-ended Members	Model Type	Plan Age	Profit Status	Qual Status
OREGON *(Cont'd)*						
Portland, OR						
Health Maintenance of Oregon	42,684		IPA	2	P	FQ
Kaiser Fdn. Health Plan of the Northwest	375,878[a]		Group	44	NP	FQ
PacifiCare of Oregon [Tigard]	62,352		Network	5	P	FQ
Physicians Assn. of Clackamas County [Clackamas]	29,132		IPA	51	NP	FQ
Qual-Med Oregon Health Plan, Inc.	32,032	8,536	IPA	4	P	FQ
Sisters of Providence Good Health Plan of OR	45,845	1,727	IPA	5	NP	FQ
Salem, OR						
Capitol Health Care	60,005[h]		IPA	12	NP	FQ
PENNSYLVANIA						
Beaver County, PA						
Riverside Health Plan [Bridgewater]	13,856		IPA	3	P	NFQ

Erie, PA

Independent Health of Pennsylvania	9,685		IPA	4	P	FQ

Harrisburg-Lebanon-Carlisle, PA

| Keystone Health Plan Central [Camp Hill] | 60,000 | | IPA | 7 | P | NFQ |

Lancaster, PA

| HealthGuard of Lancaster | 29,065 | | Network | 5 | P | FQ |

Philadelphia, PA-NJ

CIGNA Healthplan of Pennsylvania [Lester]	2,050	4,421	IPA	2	P	FQ
Delaware Valley HMO [Concordville]	130,000		IPA	11	P	FQ
Freedom Health Care, Inc. [Wayne]	27,847[c]		Network	3	P	NFQ
Greater Atlantic Health Service	49,000		Network	15	P	FQ
Group Health Partnership	25,009		Staff	15	P	FQ
HMO of Pennsylvania [Blue Bell]	542,000[a]		IPA	13	P	FQ
Keystone Health Plan East [Bala Cynwyd]	105,141		IPA	2	P	FQ
PARTNERS Health Plan - Aetna [Bala Cynwyd]	9,951		IPA	3	P	NFQ

STATE HMO Metro Location Plan Name [Headquarters City]	Pure Members	Open-ended Members	Model Type	Plan Age	Profit Status	Qual Status
PENNSYLVANIA *(Cont'd)*						
Philadelphia, PA-NJ *(Cont'd)*						
PruCare of Philadelphia [Horsham]	9,125		IPA	2	P	FQ
Vista Health Plan [King of Prussia]	22,133		IPA	3	P	NFQ
Pittsburgh, PA						
Central Medical Health Plan	13,528[i]		IPA	15	NP	NFQ
HealthAmerica PA	152,152[b]		Mixed[r]	14	P	FQ
Keystone Health Plan West, Inc.	53,057		IPA	3	P	FQ
PARTNERS Health Plan of Western PA - Aetna	20,021		IPA	3	P	FQ
Scranton-Wilkes-Barre, PA						
HMO of Northeastern PA	23,088		IPA	3	NP	FQ
Non-Metropolitan						
Geisinger Health Plan [Danville]	88,035		Group	17	NP	FQ

RHODE ISLAND

Providence, RI

HMO Rhode Island	13,505	63	IPA	3	P	FQ
MetLife HealthCare Network of RI, Inc. [Warwick]	759		IPA	2	P	NFQ
Ocean State Physician's Health Plan [Warwick]	111,846	16,527	IPA	7	P	FQ
Rhode Island Group Health Association	79,749		Staff	18	NP	FQ

SOUTH CAROLINA

Charleston, SC

Healthsource South Carolina	16,000	IPA	2	P	FQ

Columbia, SC

Companion HealthCare Corporation	27,305		IPA	5	P	FQ
Physicians Health Plan of South Carolina	8,800	3,900	IPA	4	NP	NFQ

Greenville-Spartanburg, SC

Maxicare South Carolina	15,000	Network[y]	14	P	FQ

As of 07/01/90

STATE HMO Metro Location Plan Name [Headquarters City]	Pure Members	Open-ended Members	Model Type	Plan Age	Profit Status	Qual Status
SOUTH DAKOTA						
Sioux Falls, SD						
DakotaCare	23,683		IPA	3	P	NFQ
TENNESSEE						
Chattanooga, TN-GA						
CareChoice	15,674		IPA	5	P	NFQ
Knoxville, TN						
Tennessee First Health Plan	11,719	395	IPA	3	P	NFQ
Memphis, TN-AR-MS						
EQUICOR Healthplan, Inc.	17,734[k]		IPA	2	P	NFQ
PruCare of Memphis	32,509		Group	9	P	FQ
The Apple Plan	31,000	5,500	IPA	9	NP	FQ
Nashville, TN						
EQUICOR, Inc. [Brentwood]	18,521		IPA	4	P	NFQ

Plan			Model			
PARTNERS Hlth Pln of TN/HealthMaster - Aetna	8,573	5,487	IPA	5	P	NFQ
PruCare of Nashville	28,379		Group	9	P	FQ
Tennessee Primary Care Network	19,492		Network	4	NP	NFQ

TEXAS

Amarillo, TX

First Care	26,320		IPA	3	P	FQ

Austin, TX

PCA Health Plans of Texas, Inc.*	78,723		IPA	8	P	FQ
PruCare of Austin	55,449		Group	9	P	FQ
Travelers Health Network of Austin, Inc.	26,476		IPA	4	P	FQ

Corpus Christi, TX

Coastal Bend Health Plan	21,200		IPA	4	P	FQ
Humana Health Plan of Corpus Christi	33,477[a]		IPA	7	P	FQ

Dallas, TX

CIGNA Healthplan of Texas, Inc.-Dallas Div. [Irving]	55,307	6,307	Mixed[r]	9	P	FQ
Kaiser Foundation Health Plan of Texas	115,372[a]		Group	10	NP	FQ
MetLife HealthCare Network of Texas, Inc. [Irving]	26,351		IPA	2	P	NFQ

As of 07/01/90

STATE HMO Metro Location Plan Name [Headquarters City]	Pure Members	Open-ended Members	Model Type	Plan Age	Profit Status	Qual Status
TEXAS *(Cont'd)*						
Dallas, TX *(Cont'd)*						
PruCare of North Texas	14,822		IPA	3	P	FQ
Sanus Texas Health Plan [Irving]	90,614	26,489	IPA	5	P	FQ
Southwest, an Aetna Health Plan - Aetna	51,091		IPA	4	P	FQ
Travelers Health Network of Texas, Inc. [Richardson]	4,740		IPA	3	P	NFQ
El Paso, TX						
Rio Grande HMO, Inc.	10,283		IPA	3	P	FQ
Fort Worth-Arlington, TX						
Harris Methodist Health Plan	49,600		IPA	3	NP	FQ
Houston, TX						
American General Health Plan, Inc.	850		IPA	<1	P	NFQ
CIGNA Healthplan of Texas - Houston	21,250	3,245	Mixed[t]	7	P	FQ
PARTNERS National Health Plans - Aetna	15,054		IPA	2	P	NFQ

Plan			Model			
PruCare of Houston	120,189		Group	15	P	FQ
Sanus Texas Health Plan	138,502	76,257	IPA	5	P	FQ
Travelers Health Network of Texas, Inc.	4,370		IPA	4	P	FQ
Killeen-Temple, TX						
Scott and White Health Plan	65,500		Group	8	NP	FQ
San Antonio, TX						
Humana Health Plan of San Antonio	85,950[a]		IPA	5	P	FQ
PacifiCare of Texas	36,097		Group	3	P	FQ
PruCare of San Antonio	13,994		IPA	5	P	FQ
Travelers Health Network of Texas, Inc.	6,344		IPA	4	P	FQ
UTAH						
Salt Lake City-Ogden, UT						
Educators Health Care [Murray]	0	3,155	Network	10	NP	NFQ
FHP, Inc.	120,309		Staff	15	P	FQ
HealthWise	33,238		Network	8	P	FQ
IHC Care	43,900	17,000	IPA	4	NP	FQ
Physicians Health Plan of Utah	26,558	3,784	IPA	5	P	FQ

As of 07/01/90

STATE HMO Metro Location Plan Name [Headquarters City]	Pure Members	Open-ended Members	Model Type	Plan Age	Profit Status	Qual Status
UTAH *(Cont'd)*						
Non-Metropolitan						
EQUICOR Health Plan of Utah, Inc.* [Murray]	13,616		IPA	3	P	NFQ
VERMONT						
Burlington, VT						
Community Health Plan of Vermont - CHP	36,570		Network	6	NP	FQ
VIRGINIA						
Norfolk-Virginia Beach-Newport News, VA						
EQUICOR, Inc. (Hampton Road/VA Beach)*	15,455		IPA	5	P	FQ
Optima Health Plan	55,713		IPA	5	NP	FQ
Sentara Health Plans, Inc.	43,795c		Staff	5	P	NFQ
Travelers Health Network, Inc.	9,108		IPA	5	P	FQ
Richmond-Petersburg, VA						
EQUICOR, Inc. (Richmond) [Glen Allen]	41,517		IPA	5	P	FQ

HealthKeepers of Virginia, Inc	15,655		IPA	3	P	NFQ
HMO Virginia, Inc.	26,149		IPA	5	P	FQ
PruCare of Richmond	21,296		Group	7	P	FQ
Southern Health Services	27,799		IPA	4	P	FQ

Washington, DC-MD-VA

CapitalCare [Tyson's Corner]	59,896	10,911	IPA	4	P	FQ
Choice Healthcare Plan - Aetna [Fairfax]	2,934		IPA	6	P	NFQ
PARTNERS Hlth Plans of the Mid Atlantic-Aetna [Fairfax]	40,052		IPA	6	P	FQ
Physicians Care First [Arlington]	15,122[c]		IPA	4	P	FQ

WASHINGTON

Seattle, WA

CIGNA Healthplan of Washington, Inc.	2,880	436	IPA	4	P	NFQ
Good Health Plan of Washington	20,450		IPA	2	NP	NFQ
Group Health Cooperative of Puget Sound	456,000[n]		Staff[g]	43	NP	NFQ
HealthPlus	75,653		Network	8	NP	NFQ

As of 07/01/90

STATE HMO Metro Location Plan Name [Headquarters City]	Pure Members	Open-ended Members	Model Type	Plan Age	Profit Status	Qual Status
WASHINGTON *(Cont'd)*						
Seattle, WA *(Cont'd)*						
HMO Washington	15,820		IPA	3	P	NFQ
Pacific Health	19,805		IPA	4	NP	NFQ
Qual-Med Washington Health Plan, Inc.* [Bellevue]	71,469		IPA	4	P	FQ
Virginia Mason Health Plan - Aetna	34,513		Network	4	P	NFQ
WEST VIRGINIA						
Wheeling, WV-OH						
Health Plan of the Upper Ohio Valley [St. Clairsville]	72,295		IPA	10	NP	FQ
WISCONSIN						
Appleton-Oshkosh-Neenah, WI						
Network Health Plan - Aetna	24,130		Network	6	P	NFQ
United Health of Wisconsin Ins. Co., Inc.	17,300		IPA	2	P	NFQ

Eau Claire, WI

Eau Claire-Chippewa Health Protection Plan [Wausau]	539	5,162	IPA	15	P	NFQ
Group Health Cooperative of Eau Claire [Altoona]	15,349		Staff	13	NP	NFQ
Midelfort Health Plan	22,292		Network	8	P	NFQ

Green Bay, WI

Employer's Health Care Plan	30,271[c]		Network	5	P	NFQ
Green Bay Health Protection Plan [Wausau]	19,173		IPA	17	P	NFQ

La Crosse, WI

Greater LaCrosse Health Plans, Inc. [LaCrosse]	4,498		Group	3	P	NFQ

Madison, WI

Allhealth	3,100[b]		IPA	4	NP	NFQ
DeanCare HMO [Middleton]	106,883		Network	6	P	FQ
Group Health Cooperative of So. Central WI	34,543		Staff	13	NP	FQ
Physicians Plus HMO	58,565		Network	6	P	NFQ
Q Care	10,737[b]		IPA	7	NP	NFQ
U-Care HMO, Inc.	14,737		IPA	1	NP	NFQ

STATE HMO Metro Location Plan Name [Headquarters City]	Pure Members	Open-ended Members	Model Type	Plan Age	Profit Status	Qual Status
WISCONSIN *(Cont'd)*						
Milwaukee, WI						
CHOICE Healthcare Plan - Aetna	10,589		IPA	4	P	NFQ
Compcare Health Services Insurance Corp.	152,302		Network	18	P	FQ
Family Health Plan	84,423		Staff	10	NP	FQ
Maxicare Health Insurance Company	21,000		IPA	8	P	FQ
MetLife HealthCare Network of Wisconsin, Inc.	2,622		IPA	2	P	NFQ
PrimeCare Health Plan	99,500		IPA	6	P	NFQ
Samaritan Health Plan	74,680		IPA	8	P	FQ
Wisconsin Health Organization Insurance Corp.	114,201		IPA	4	P	FQ
Minneapolis/St. Paul, MN-WI						
HMO Midwest [Hudson]	8,982		Network	5	NP	NFQ

Wausau, WI

North Central Health Protection Plan	26,259	3,352	IPA	18	NP	NFQ
Oshkosh Area Health Protection Plan	3,430		IPA	1	P	NFQ

Non-Metropolitan

Greater WI Rapids Health Protection Plan [Wausau]	632[m]		IPA	10	P	NFQ
HMO of Wisconsin Insurance Corporation [Prarie Du Sac]	36,946		IPA	6	P	NFQ
Security Health Plan of Wisconsin, Inc. [Marshfield]	59,905		Network	18	NP	NFQ

Appendix C

TREATMENT SUMMARY

SUBSCRIBER INFORMATION

Name: _____ D.O.B. _____

Address: _____

Employer: _____ Insurance: _____

Subscriber: _____ Group Number: _____

PATIENT INFORMATION: (if different from subscriber)

Name: _____ D.O.B. _____

Address: _____

Primary Care Physician: _____

ASSESSMENT/DIAGNOSIS INFORMATION:

A.   Current symptoms and impairment in social/occupational functioning:

_____

_____

_____

_____

_____

_____

_____

B. Use of mood-altering substances, including alcohol or other illicit drugs and family history of same. Indicate if problematic:

_____
_____
_____
_____
_____
_____

C. Present prescribed medication for medical or psychiatric condition:

_____
_____
_____

Is there need for evaluation for medication, psychological testing or physician evaluation?

_____ yes   _____ no

If YES, explain: _____

_____

D. DSM III-R Diagnosis (include code)

Axis 1: _____
Axis 2: _____
Axis 3: _____
Axis 4: _____
Axis 5: _____

307

TREATMENT PLAN:

A. Objective of Treatment: _____

B. Interventions; (refer to the following as relevant: theme of focus of sessions, techniques to be used, assignments outside therapy, use of community resources, use of chemotherapy)

_____
_____
_____
_____
_____
_____
_____

C. Mode of treatment (i.e., group, individual, etc.) _____

D. Frequency of sessions: _____   Length of sessions: _____

E. Number of sessions already conducted (this enrollment year) _____

F. Estimated number sessions needed to complete objectives: _____

PERSON PROVIDING TREATMENT: (Print) _____

Signature: _____   Date: _____

MCC Companies, Inc.

Treatment Update

Patient Name: _____ DOB: _____

Describe response to treatment: (achievement of or progress toward treatment goals):

_____

_____

_____

Number of sessions previously authorized by MCC: _____

Number of sessions completed to date: _____

Number of additional sessions requested: _____

Frequency of sessions: _____

Current DSM III-R Diagnosis: _____

Current Symptoms: _____

_____

Modification to treatment goals: _____

_____

Rationale for additional sessions: _____

_____

Name of Therapist: _____

Signature: _____ Date: _____

MCC Companies, Inc.
7702 Parham Road, Suite 104
Richmond, VA 23294
(804) 747-MCC2

310

MCC Companies, Inc.

Closing Summary

PATIENT'S NAME: _____   DATE OF CLOSING: _____

DATE OF BIRTH: _____

   I. **Extent of Contact**

A) Client seen from _____ to _____

B) Number of appointments _____

C) Number of "no shows" or cancelled appointments _____

  II. **Presenting Problems**

_____

_____

_____

  III. **Brief Description of Course of Treatment**

_____

_____

_____

IV. __Reason for Closing__

V. Diagnosis at End of Treatment, Prognosis an/or Recommendations.

Signature: _____

Title: _____

Return to: **MCC Companies, Inc., 7702 Parham Rd., Ste. 104, Richmond, VA 23294, Attn: Medical Records Dept.**

_____

_____

_____

RE: _____

Dear _____:

This patient was seen for an evaluation on _____. Our
Intake Team has carefully evaluated this patient and determined that
the primary diagnosis is _____

_____.

We are referring this patient to you for
_____ therapy and have identified the treatment goals as:

1. _____

2. _____

3. _____

313

visits are authorized and we believe these will be sufficient to resolve the patient's presenting problem. If you have any addition or disagreement to these treatment goals, or number of sessions authorized, please submit a written diagnostic report and treatment summary by the fourth visit. On completion or termination of treatment, for any reason, please submit the enclosed closing treatment summary.

The MCC case manager is _____.

Cordially yours,

Norman Winegar, L.C.S.W., C.E.A.P
Executive Director

Appendix D

S.O.A.P PROCESS NOTE RECORDING FORMAT

S (Subjective)

- What the patient says
- Basic history (first session)
- Major focus of session — content

O (Objective)

- Mental status exam
- Appearance
- Speech
- Nonverbal behavior
- Defenses

A (Assessment)

- 5 axis diagnosis DSM-III-R (initial session)
- Subsequent sessions:
  - Improvement vs. regression
  - Motivation
  - Relapse behavior

P (Plan)

- Any further assessment needed
- Use of community resources
- Homework
- Goals of treatment
- Spacing of sessions
- Contract for length of treatment
- Development of support systems
- Techniques to be used

Appendix E

Important Managed Mental Health Care / Employee Assistance Program Companies

NAME	ADDRESS	Parentage
American Biodyne, Inc.	400 Oyster Point Blvd. Suite 306 S. San Francisco, CA 94080 (415) 742-0802 Albert Waxman, Ph D President Nicholas Cummings, Ph D CEO	Independent
American Psych Management, Inc. (APM)	1560 Wilson Blvd. Suite 1000 Arlington, VA 22209 (703) 528-2255 John Hill Acting CEO	Value Health
TAO	1901 Market Street 32nd Floor P.O. Box 15988 Philadelphia, PA 19103 (215) 241-2400 Anthony Panzetta CEO	BCBS
Human Management Strategies (HMS)	1725 Duke Street, Ste. 300 Alexandria, VA 22314 (800) 553-8700 (703) 838-8400 Seton Shields President	BCBS
Lifeplus	Lifeplus Plaza 6441 Coldwater Canyon Ave N. Hollywood, CA 91606 (818) 769-3915 Ed Mullen CEO	Pacificare

Personnel Performance Consultants, Inc. (PPC)	1401 S. Brentwood Blvd. Suite 400 St. Louis, MO 63144 (800) 821-0055	Independent
	Carl Tisone CEO	
Human Affairs International, Inc. (HAI)	5801 South Fashion Blvd. Murray, Utah 84107 (800) 999-4241	AETNA
	Jim Plack, CEO	
Managed Health Network, Inc.(MHN)	5100 West Goldleaf Circle Suite 300 Los Angeles, CA 90056 (213) 299-0999	Independent
	Ron Morelan, CEO	
United Behavioral Systems, Inc. (UBS)	3600 W. 80th Street Ste. 210 Minneapolis, MN 55431 (612) 832-3300 Jack Newstrom President and CEO	United Health Care
Preferred Health Care	Post Office Box 787 Wilton, CT 06897 (800) 433-8565	Four Winds Hospital
	David McDonnell CEO	
MCC Companies, Inc.	11095 Viking Drive Suite 350 Eden Prairie, MN 55344 (612) 943-9500 (800) 433-5768	CIGNA
	Travers Wills President	

Appendix F

BRIEF THERAPY READING LIST

Bennett, M. J., & Wisneski, M. J. (1979). Continuous psychotherapy within an HMO. *American Journal of Psychiatry, 136*, 1283-1287.

Bennett, M. (1984). Brief Psychotherapy and Adult Development. *Psychotherapy, 2*, 171-177.

Budman, S. H., & Bennett, M. J. (1983). Short-term group psychotherapy. In H. Kaplan & B. Sadock (Eds.), *Comprehensive group psychotherapy* (rev. ed., pp. 138-144). Baltimore: Williams & Williams.

Budman, S. H., & Clifford, M. (1979). Short-term group therapy for couples in a health maintenance organization. *Professional Psychology: Research and Practice, 10*, 419-429.

Budman, S. H., & Gurman, A. S. (1983). The practice of brief therapy. *Professional Psychology: Research and Practice, 14*, 277-292.

Budman, S. H., & Gurman, A. S. (1988). *Theory and Practice of Brief Therapy*. New York: Guilford Press.

Davanloo, H. (Ed.). (1978a). *Basic principles and techniques in short-term dynamic psychotherapy*. New York: Spectrum.

Davanloo, H. (1980). A method of short-term dynamic psychotherapy. In H. Davanloo (Ed.), *Short-term dynamic psychotherapy* (pp. 43-71). New York: Jason Aronson.

De Shazer, S. (1982). *Patterns of brief therapy*. New York: Guilford Press.

De Shazer, S. (1985). *Keys to solution in brief therapy*. New York: Norton.

De Shazer, S. (1988). *Clues: Investigating solutions in brief therapy*. New York: Norton.

Fisch, R., Weakland, J. H., & Segal, L. (1982). *The tactics of change: Doing therapy briefly*. San Francisco: Jossey-Bass.

Flegenheimer, W. V. (1982). *Techniques of brief psychotherapy*. New York: Jason Aronson.

Haley, J. (1973). *Uncommon therapy: The psychiatric techniques of Milton H. Erickson, M.D.* New York: Norton.

Haley, J. (1976). *Problem solving therapy*. San Francisco: Jossey-Bass.

Koss, M. P., et al. (1988). Brief Psychotherapy Methods in Clinical Research. *Journal of Consulting and Clinical Psychology*, *54*, 60-67.

Madanes, C. (1981). *Strategic family therapy*. San Francisco: Jossey-Bass.

Mann, J. (1973). *Time-limited psychotherapy*. Cambridge, MA: Harvard University Press.

Mann, J., & Goldman, R. (1982). *A casebook in time-limited psychotherapy*. New York: McGraw-Hill.

O'Hanlon, W. H. (1987). Taproots: *Underlying principles of Milton Erickson's therapy and hypnosis*. New York: Norton.

O'Hanlon, W. H., & Weiner-Davis, M. (1989). *In search of solutions: A new direction in psychotherapy*. New York: Norton.

Parad, H. J., & Parad, L. G. (1968). A study of crisis oriented planned short-term treatment: Part I. *Social Casework*, *49*, 346-355.

Parad, L. G., & Parad, H. J. (1968). A study of crisis oriented planned short-term treatment: Part II. *Social Casework*, *49*, 418-426.

Pekarik, G. (1989). *Brief Therapy Training Manual*. Unpublished manuscript.

Sifneos, P. E. (1979). *Short-term dynamic psychotherapy: Evaluation and technique*. New York: Plenum Press.

Small, L. (1979). *The briefer psychotherapies*. New York: Brunner/Mazel.

Talmon, M. (1990). *Single Session Therapy*. San Francisco: Jossey-Bass.

Watzlawick, P., Fisch, R., & Segal, L. (1982). *The tactics of change*. San Francisco: Jossey-Bass.

Weakland, J. H., Fisch, R., Watzlawick, P., & Bodin, A. (1974). Brief therapy: Focused problem resolution. *Family Process*, *13*, 141-168.

Wells, R. H., & Giannetti, V. J. (Ed.) (1990). *Handbook of the Brief Psychotherapies*. New York: Plenum Publishing Corporation.

Wolberg, L. R. (1980). *Handbooks of short-term psychotherapy*. New York: Grune & Stratton.

Developed by, and provided courtesy of Dr. John Bistline.

Resource Directory

GOVERNMENT

Department of Commerce
Main Commerce Building
14th E. Constitution Ave., NW
Washington, DC 20230
(202) 377-2000

Department of Health & Human Services
200 Independence Ave.
Washington, DC 20201
(202) 619-0287

Department of Labor
200 Constitution Ave NW
Washington, DC 20210
(202) 523-6666

Health Care Financing Administration
6325 Security Boulevard
Baltimore, MD 21207
(301) 966-3000

National Center for Health Services Research
and Health Care Technology Assessment
Parklawn Building
5600 Fishers Lane
Rockville, MD 20857
(301) 443-4100

National Center for Health Statistics
3700 East-West Highway
Hyattsville, MD 20782
(301) 436-8500

National Health Information Clearinghouse
P.O. Box 1133
Washington, DC 20013
(800) 336-4797

National Institutes of Health
9000 Rockville Pike
Bethesda, MD 20892
(301) 496-4000

National Technical Information Service
5285 Port Rogal Road
Springfield, VA 22161
(703) 487-4650

PROFESSIONAL ASSOCIATIONS
AND OTHER ORGANIZATIONS

American Association for Marriage and Family Therapy
1100 17th St., NW
10th Floor
Washington, DC 20036
(202) 452-0109

American Association of Preferred Provider Organizations
Suite 600
111 E. Wacker Dr.
Chicago, IL 60610
(312) 644-6610

American Insurance Association
Suite 1000
1130 Connecticut Ave., NW
Washington, DC 20036
(202) 828-7100

American Managed Care and Review Association
1227 25th St. NW
Suite 610
Washington, DC 20037
(202) 728-0506

American Mental Health Counselors Association
5999 Stevenson Ave.
Alexandria, VA 22304
(800) 326-2642

American Nursing Association
2420 Pershing Road
Kansas City, MO 64108
(816) 474-5720

American Psychiatric Association
1400 K Street, NW
Washington, DC 20005
(202) 682-6070

Blue Cross and Blue Shield Association
676 N. St. Clair
Chicago, IL 60611
(312) 440-6000

Employee Assistance Professionals Association
Suite 1001
4601 N. Fairfax Drive
Arlington, VA 22203
(703) 522-6272

Group Health Association of America
Suite 600
1129 Twentieth St., NW
Washington, DC 20036
(202) 778-3200

Health Insurance Association of America
1025 Connecticut Ave., NW
Washington, DC 20036
(202) 223-7780

Institute for a Drug-Free Workplace
P.O. Box 65708
Washington, DC 20035-5708
(202) 463-5530

InterStudy
Center for Managed Care Research
5715 Christmas Lake Road
P.O. Box 458
Excelsior, MN 55331-0458
(612) 474-1176

Joint Commission on Accreditation of Healthcare Organizations
One Renaissance Blvd
Oakbrook Terrace, IL 60181
(708) 916-5600

National Association of Private Psychiatric Hospitals
Suite 1000
1319 F St., NW
Washington, DC 20004
(202) 393-6700

National Association of Social Workers
7981 Eastern Ave
Silver Spring, MD 20910
(800) 638-8799

National Council on Alcoholism and Drug Dependence
12 West 21st St.
New York, NY 10010
(212) 206-6700

National Employee Benefits Institute
Suite 400
2445 M. Street, NW
Washington, DC 20037
(800) 558-7258

National Federation of Societies for Clinical Social Work
P.O. Box 3740
Arlington, VA 22203
(708) 998-1680

New York Business Group on Health
622 Third Ave
New York, NY 10017
(212) 808-0550

Self Insurance Institute of America
P.O. Box 15466
Santa Ana, CA 92705
(714) 261-2553

Society for Human Resource Management
   (formerly the American Society for Personal Administration)
606 N. Washington St.
Alexandria, VA 22314
(703) 548-3440

U.S. Chamber of Commerce
1615 H St., NW
Washington, DC 20062
(202) 659-6000

Washington Business Group on Health
Suite 800
777 N. Capitol St., NE
Washington, DC 20002
(202) 408-9320

Glossary

Carve-Outs: A benefit strategy in which an employer separates ("carves out") the mental health and substance abuse portion of health care benefits from others and hires a MMHC company to manage or provide these benefits through its networks. Affords the employer with specialized management for this portion of the overall benefits package.

Community Rating: A premium rating methodology frequently used by HMOs. The HMO using this method must charge the same amount of money per member for all members of a plan. The methodology does not allow for employer account-specific variables to influence pricing. Contrasts with Experience Rating.

Cost of Services Ratio (COS Ratio): The ratio between the cost incurred by the managed care entity that is directly related to service delivery, and the amount of revenue taken in. A COS ratio of 75% or more is common in MMHC operations, and excludes administrative or overhead costs.

Current Procedural Terminology (CPT) Codes: Sets of five-digit codes frequently used for billing professional services.

Employee Assistance Program: An employer-sponsored counseling and consultation service aimed at assisting employees or family members experiencing emotional, substance abuse, family, or other problems that can interfere with productivity or worker safety. EAPs pursue goals by ensuring the provision of appropriate and cost-effective services.

EAPs may be offered by employers as an integral part of the benefit plan, or as an entirely separate program. The EAP may be voluntary or mandatory. In mandatory EAPs the benefit plan reimburses only care that is delivered by a clinician associated with the EAP's provider network. Incentivized EAPs feature a higher level of reimbursement when care is rendered by a member of the EAP provider network. In addition to provider networks, EAPs may also offer utilization management and other managed care functions.

Enrollee: An individual who is eligible for benefits under a health care plan. Frequently used in connection with indemnity insurance.

Experience Rating: A premium rating methodology that adjusts an account's rate based on the utilization experience and other factors specific to the account. This system allows for lower premiums for employers who have healthy workforces, and contrasts with Community Rating methodology which averages data for multiple groups of employees.

Fiduciary: Under ERISA, any person or entity that exercises discretionary control over the administration of a benefit plan. Self-insured employers can delegate this responsibility to MMHC or UR firms concurring Mental Health and Substance Abuse benefits.

HMO Act of 1973: Amended in 1988. This law allowed HMOs to become "federally qualified" by meeting various standards. Once so designated, the HMO has the right to ask any local employer of twenty-five or more employees to offer it as a health care benefit option. HMOs were required to charge the same "community rate" to all employers, pooling all employers together for risk purposes. In 1988, Congress amended the Act. The right of HMOs to put themselves on the benefit menu of local employers was scheduled to expire in 1995. HMOs were allowed to adjust premiums by actual employer group experience, no longer adhering to a community rating system. Caps were placed in charges to smaller employer groups. HMOs were also permitted to provide services through non-HMO physicians, charging extra fees when members utilize such services.

Integrated Health Plans: A type of benefit plan in which all employees are enrolled into a single managed care system for all health care services. Members may have options to utilize nonnetwork providers, but at an increased cost.

Managed Care or Managed Mental Health Care (MMHC): Refers to any of a variety of systems and strategies aimed at marshalling appropriate clinical and financial resources to ensure needed care for consumers. It features increased structure and accountability for providers and the overall coordination of care, while eliminating duplicative or unnecessary services.

Management Information System (MIS): The computer hardware, software, and automated systems that provide support for the management of a business.

Mandated Benefits: Minimal benefit levels established by statutes enacted by state legislatures. These vary from state to state and can add to overall health care costs. ERISA exempts employers who are self-insured from these mandates. Other exceptions have been made for "basic," low cost, insurance products that can be offered to the uninsured segment of the workforce.

Medical Reimbursement Account: An increasingly popular feature of new employer sponsored health benefit plans designed to assist employees with the increased cost-sharing associated with these plans. The employee annually sets aside pre-tax dollars into the medical reimbursement account which may be used for expenses such as copayments, deductibles, eyeglasses, well baby care, or child care expenses. Employers sometimes contribute to these accounts.

Member: An individual who is eligible for benefits under a health care plan, particularly an HMO or other prepaid system.

Network or Provider Network: A group of providers, organized, accredited, and administered by a MMHC firm. Members agree to practice in an effective, cost-conscious manner utilizing the MMHC firm's clinical guidelines or standards. Members also agree to discounted fee arrangements. In turn, they are eligible for referrals, through the MMHC firm, of members of employer groups contracting with the firm. Providers agree to the MMHC firm's quality management program. The network may include both inpatient and outpatient providers. It is increasingly important for providers to join networks in order to allow access to their services by large numbers of potential patients. This requires providers to become familiar with goal-oriented, solution-focused therapies, to manage practices efficiently, and to develop innovative practice styles in order to compete successfully for referrals.

Open Enrollment Period: The time period during which an employee may change or join a health care plan. This usually occurs once per year for each employer group. Most HMOs have about half their accounts available for open enrollment in the Fall, with an effective date of January 1.

Out-of-Pocket Maximum: The maximum amount an insured person will have to pay for a covered health care expense. Often this amount is $500, $1,000, or more, or a percentage of annual salary. Usually calculated on a yearly basis.

Per Diem Reimbursement: A system used most commonly with hospitals or partial hospital programs and based on a predetermined set rate per day of care, rather than usual charges. This system is a cost containment measure, usually assuring the facility of referral volume and the managed care entity of discounted fees.

Per Employee, Per Year (PEPY): A payment method used in financing Employee Assistance Programs on a pre-paid, per capita basis.

Per Member, Per Month (PMPM): A payment method used in financing managed care arrangements under which the vendor is paid for each enrollee each month.

Practice Guidelines: Recommended therapies and procedures for the treatment of specific disorders so as to achieve optimum results as efficiently as possible. They are not rigid standards, but rather offer supportive guidance to clinicians. Many MMHC organizations use such guidelines for quality assurance or accountability purposes. Practice guidelines are developed from the clinical literature, professional societies, and/or through other clinician input forums.

Pre-Admission Review (PAR): Also known as precertification for admission. A common function in various managed care systems. This term is also commonly used to denote a "participating" facility, one that is contracted with a managed care entity to participate in its utilization management activities, including preadmission review.

Preferred Provider Arrangement (PPA): An agreement between a business entity and a provider or group of providers. Differs from a PPO, which is an actual organization.

Preferred Provider Organization (PPO): An arrangement by which an entity contracts with an organization of providers for specified services. These services are delivered on a discounted fee basis, and the providers are guaranteed a volume of referrals, prompt claims payment, etc. The providers also agree to comply with utilization management procedures.

Primary Care Physician (PCP): Usually internists, family physicians, general practitioners, and pediatricians. Some managed care plans require PCP screening and referral of members in need of mental health or substance abuse treatment services.

Provider: A professional who delivers clinical services to a managed care member. Facility provider refers to hospitals or other institutional entities.

Provider Relations Manager: A coordinating position, found in some HMOs, which has responsibility for the recruitment and credentialing of PCPs or other providers. Provider relations is a function in all managed mental health care systems which utilize Provider Networks.

Reasonable and Customary Charge: Also known as usual, customary and reasonable charge (UCR). The maximum amount an insurer will consider as eligible for reimbursement. A claims cost control device.

Utilization Management (UM) or Utilization Review (UR): Any of several techniques and procedures used to monitor and evaluate the necessity or appropriateness of care for the purposes of insurance coverage or provider reimbursement.

Index